Malaria

Edited by Fyson H. Kasenga

Published in London, United Kingdom

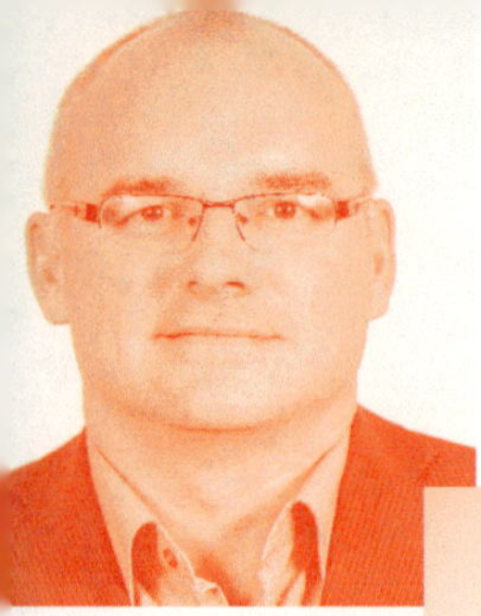
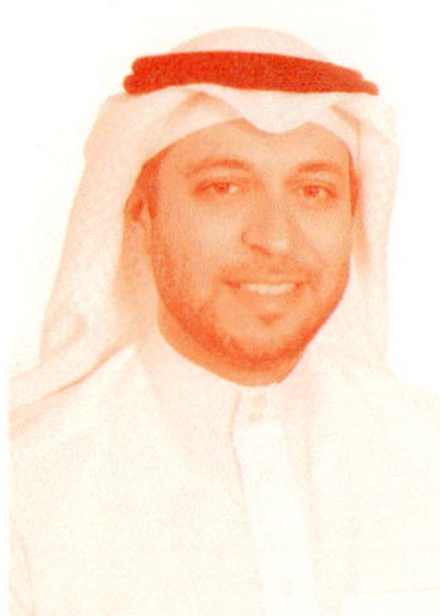
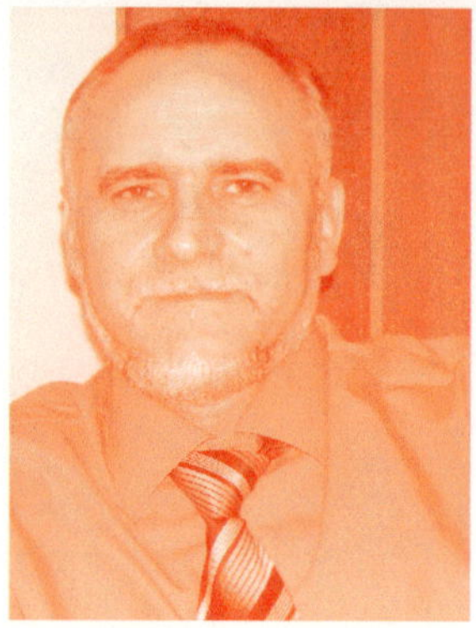
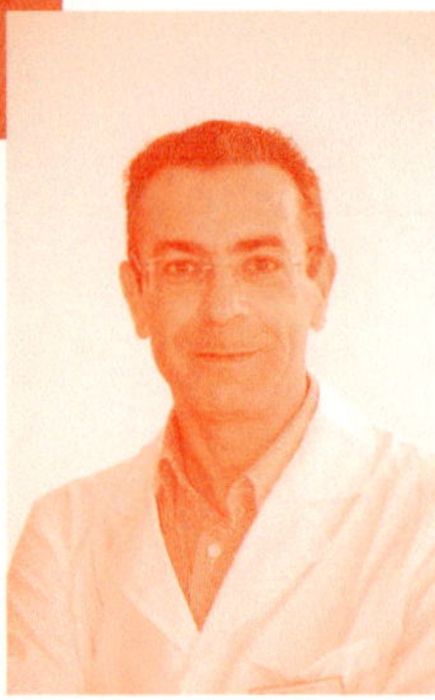
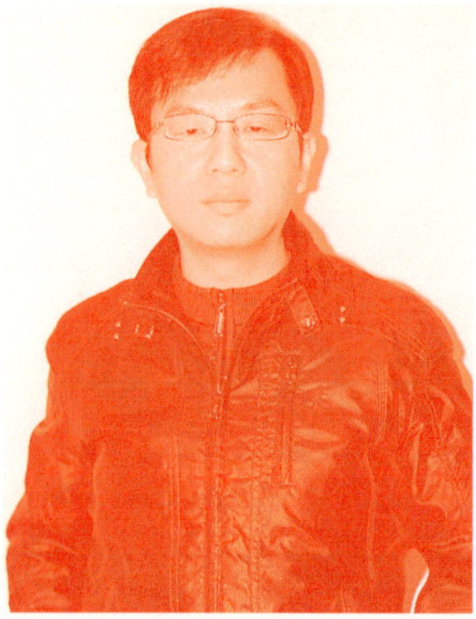
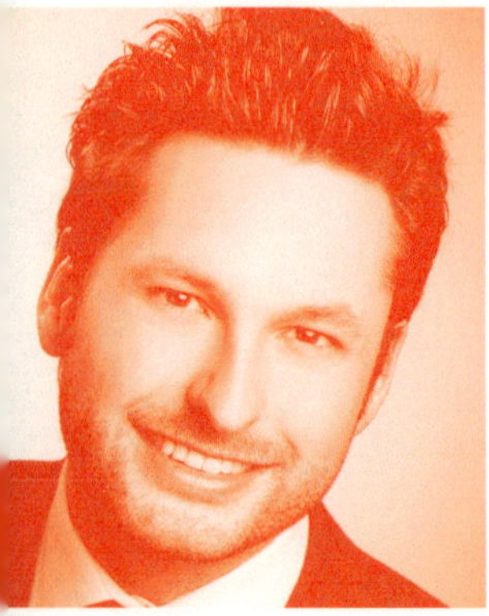
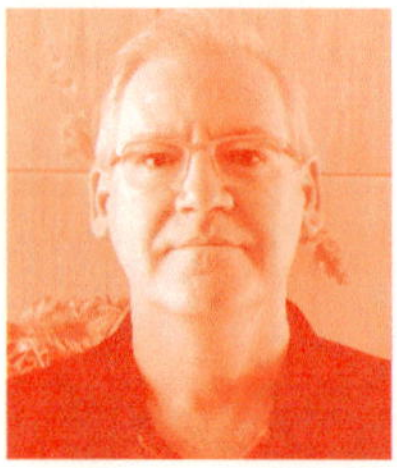

IntechOpen

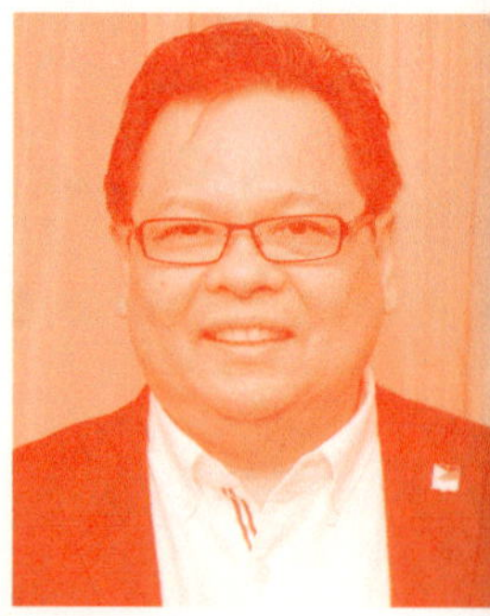
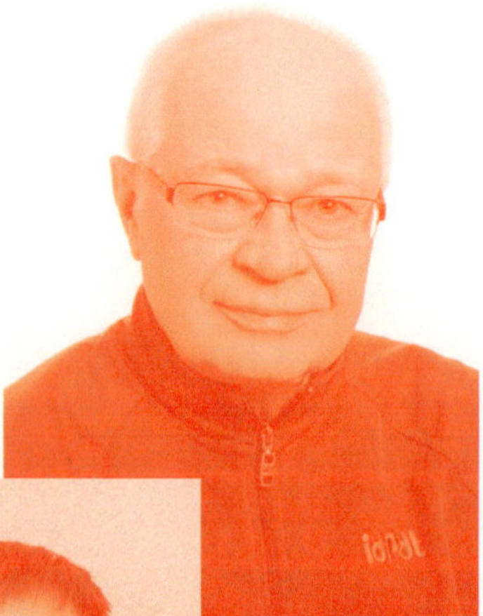
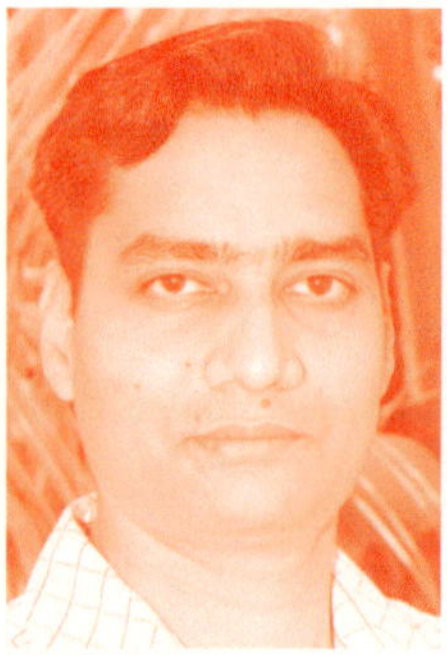
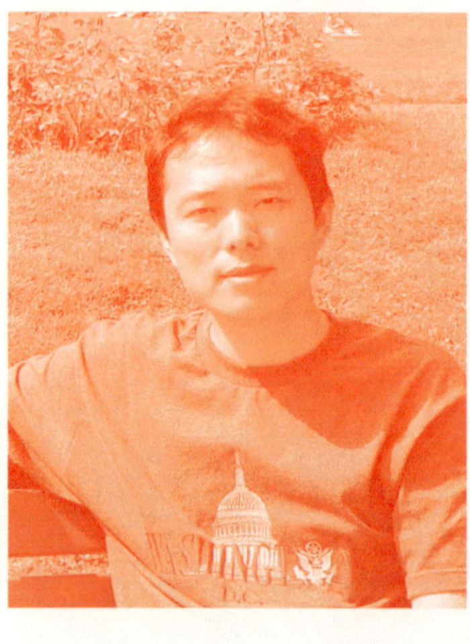
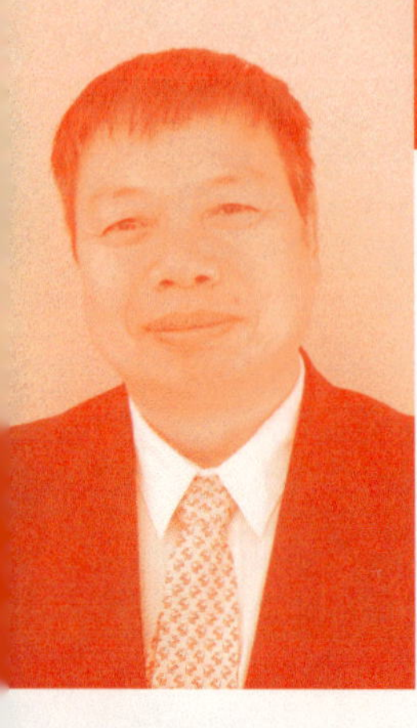
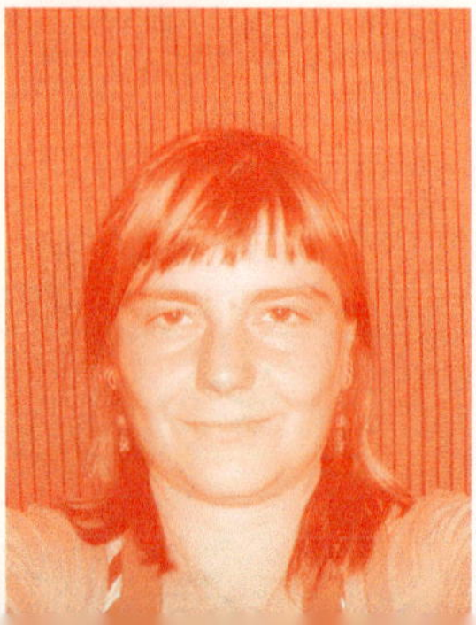

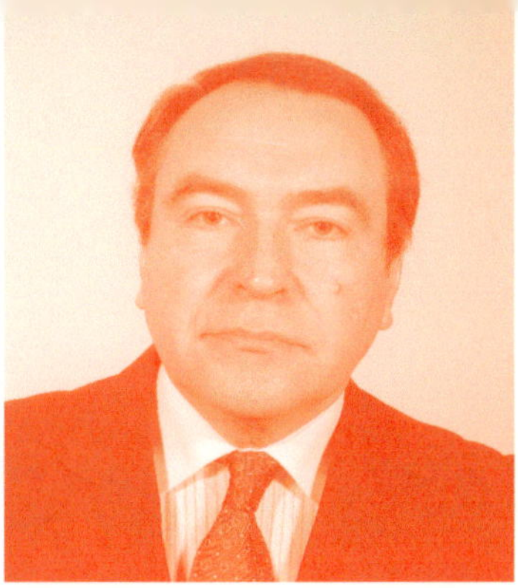
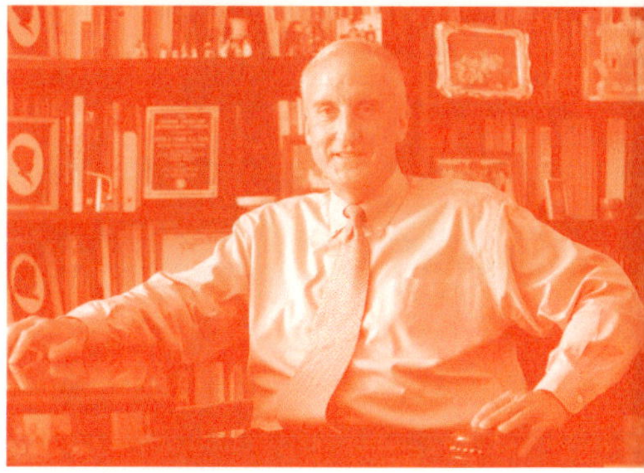
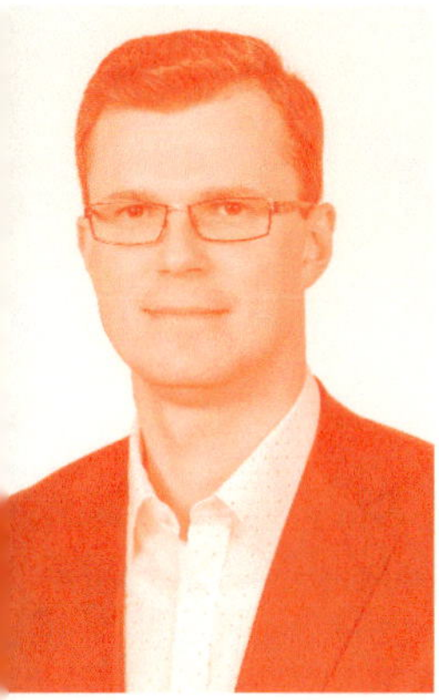
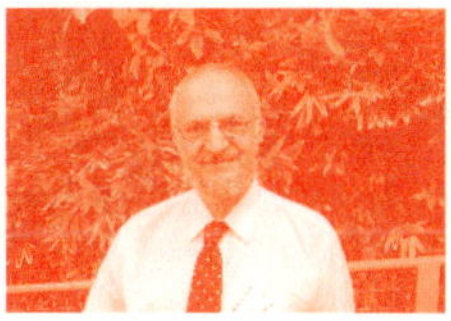
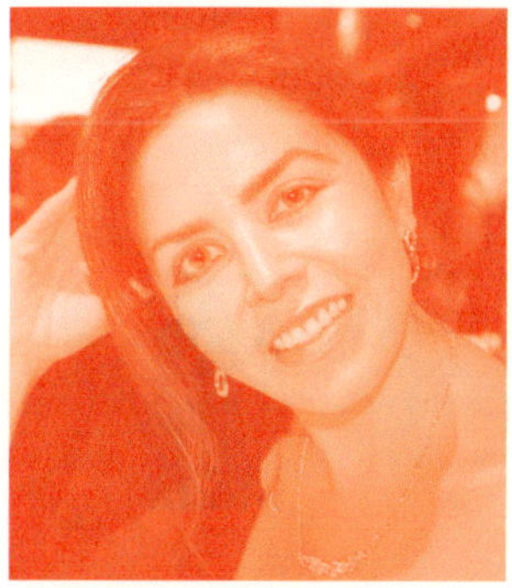

Supporting open minds since 2005

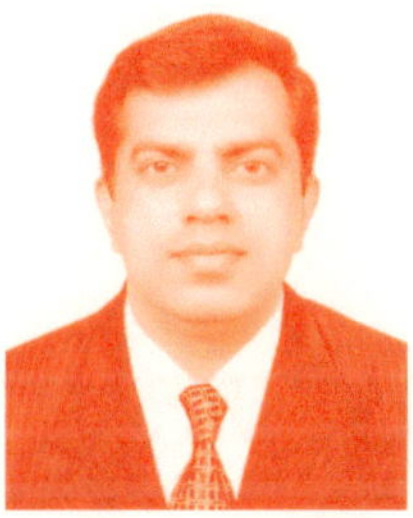
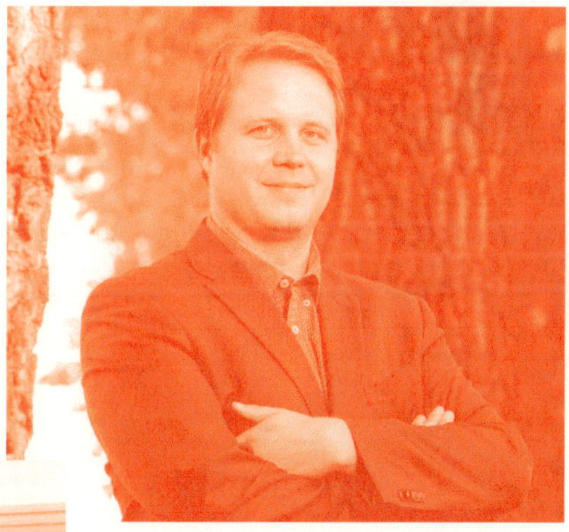
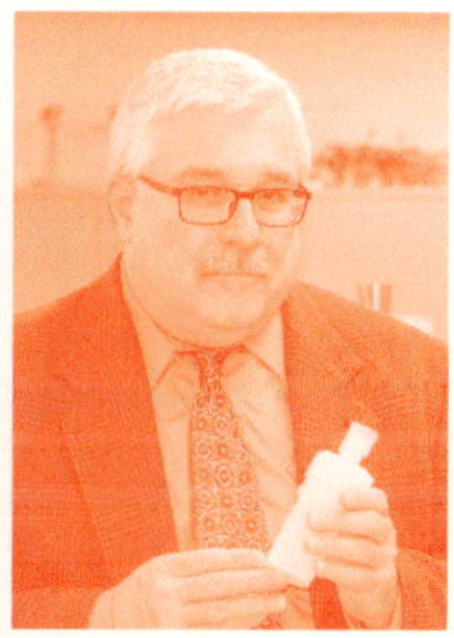
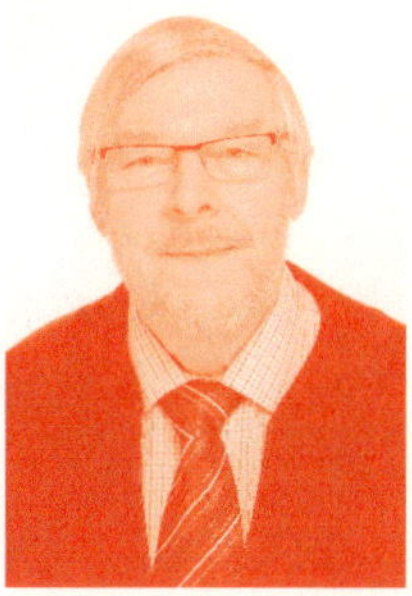
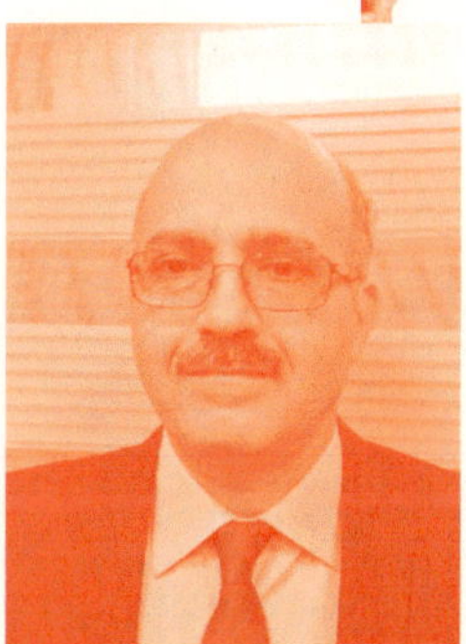
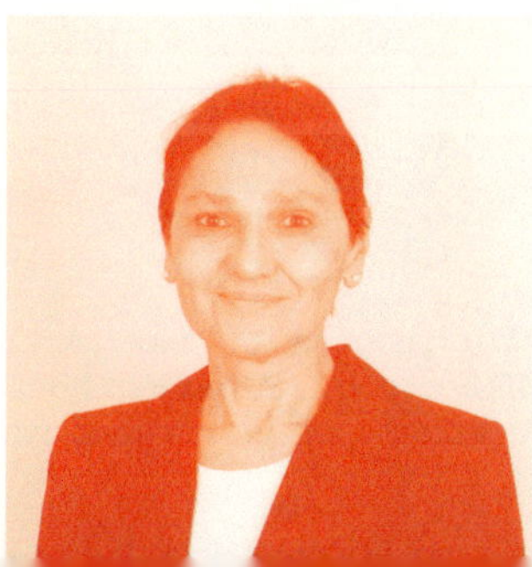
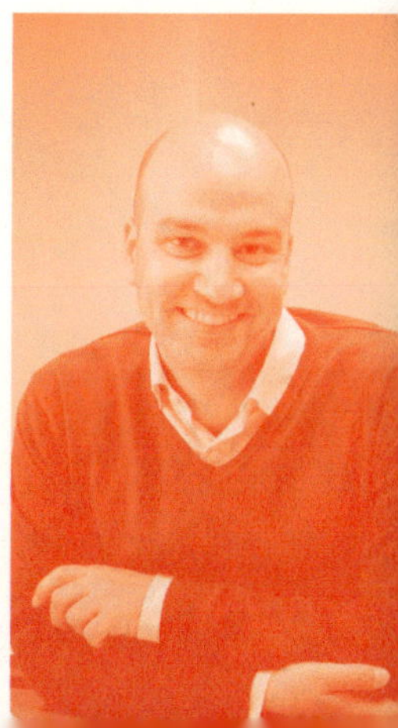

Malaria
http://dx.doi.org/10.5772/intechopen.77656
Edited by Fyson H. Kasenga

Part of IntechOpen Book Series: Infectious Diseases, Volume 4
Book Series Editor: Shailendra K. Saxena

Contributors
Hanem Fathy Khater, Kadarkarai Murugan, Nelissa P. Vaz, Marimuthu Govindarajan, Abdelfattah M. Selim, Galal A. Abouelella, Nour A. Abouelella, Alvaro E. Eiras, Kelly S. Paixão, Marcelo C. Resende, José L. Acebal, Erika M. de Carvalho, July A. H. Muñoz, Simone S. Valverde, Omolade Olayinka Okwa, Neyder Contreras-Puentes, Obadiah Moyo, Greanious Alfred Mavondo, Wisdom Peresuh, Joy Mavondo, Blessing Nkazimulo Mkhwanazi, Larson Boundenga, Qigui Li, Brandon Pybus

First published in London, United Kingdom, 2019 by IntechOpen
IntechOpen is the global imprint of INTECHOPEN LIMITED, registered in England and Wales, registration number: 11086078, 7th floor, 10 Lower Thames Street, London, EC3R 6AF, United Kingdom
Printed in Croatia

British Library Cataloguing-in-Publication Data
A catalogue record for this book is available from the British Library

Additional hard and PDF copies can be obtained from orders@intechopen.com

Malaria
Edited by Fyson H. Kasenga
p. cm.
Print ISBN 978-1-78984-121-3
Online ISBN 978-1-78984-122-0
eBook (PDF) ISBN 978-1-83968-108-0
ISSN 2631-6188

For EU product safety concerns:
IN TECH d.o.o., Prolaz Marije Krucifikse Kozulić 3, 51000 Rijeka, Croatia, info@intechopen.com or visit our website at intechopen.com.

IntechOpen Book Series

Infectious Diseases

Volume 4

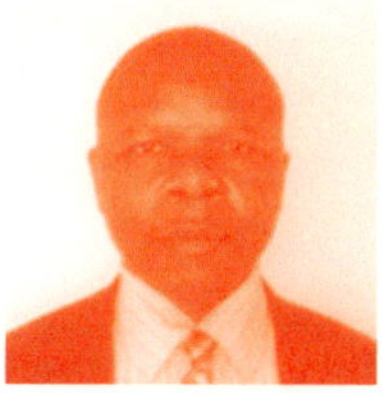

Dr. Fyson H. Kasenga is a graduate of Tumaini University, Kilimanjaro Christian Medical College, Moshi, Tanzania, and Umea University, Sweden. He obtained a Master's degree in Public Health and a PhD in Public Health and Epidemiology. He has a background in clinical medicine and has taken courses at higher diploma levels in Public Health from the University of Transkei (UNITRA), Republic of South Africa, and African Medical and Research Foundation (AMREF) in Nairobi, Kenya. Dr. Kasenga has worked in different places in and outside Malawi, and has held various positions, such as licensed medical officer, HIV/AIDS program officer, and HIV/AIDS resource person in the International Department of Diakonhjemmet College, Oslo, Norway. He also managed an Integrated HIV/AIDS Prevention Program for over 5 years. Besides working as Deputy Vice Chancellor, Malawi Adventist University, Malamulo Campus, Dr. Kasenga complements the overall vision of putting Malawi Adventist University on a world map as a "World Class University." He brings with him his expertise as a mentor for both local and international students, manages a sanitary pad-making project to keep girls in school, is a peer reviewer for several scientific papers and a researcher with more than 10 publications, and has edited several text books on HIV/AIDS-related issues, including communicable and non-communicable diseases. Dr. Kasenga has a special interest in HIV/AIDS-related issues focusing on Prevention of Mother to Child Transmission of HIV (PMTCT). Furthermore, he promotes the spirit of openness, transparency, and accountability for both academic and non-academic communities.

Editor of Volume 4:
Fyson H. Kasenga
Deputy Vice Chancellor, Malawi Adventist University
Malamulo College of Health of Sciences, Makwasa, Malawi

Book Series Editor:
Shailendra K. Saxena
King George's Medical University

Scope of the Series

The series will give a most comprehensive overview of recent trends in various infectious diseases (as per the most recent Baltimore classification), as well as general concepts of infections, immunopathology, diagnosis, treatment, epidemiology and etiology to current clinical recommendations in management of infectious diseases, highlighting the ongoing issues, recent advances, with future directions in diagnostic approaches and therapeutic strategies. This book series will focus on various aspects and properties of infectious diseases whose deep understanding is very important for safeguarding human race from more loss of resources and economies due to pathogens.

Contents

Preface

Communicable diseases are prevalent worldwide. In sub-Saharan Africa, communicable diseases cause premature and preventable deaths. Their negative effects are often felt in these poor and inadequate resource settings. Effective implementation of environmental management coupled with community involvement and participation may reduce the burden of communicable diseases, including malaria. Application of simple control and preventable measures that are culturally acceptable, affordable, accessible, and achievable may be the mainstay of dealing with this public health problem in a sustainable manner. The positive effect of successful intervention may be manifested by the reduction of disease burden among women and children, more particularly children under five years of age who die in large numbers. More often than not it is the individual's responsibility to safeguard their own health in all aspects such as positive change in lifestyles, good health-seeking behavior, and where possible control of the environment, hence the effect of climate change.

It is the view of the authors that the readers of this text book will derive maximum benefits from it, use it as a reference manual in their workplaces, and share the knowledge with the communities they serve. It is evident that change is enacted from within the mindset of an individual, then transmitted to families, communities, and eventually nations, who will change thereby create an environment better for everybody.

The book focuses on different types of malaria, more especially *Plasmodium falciparum*, which is detrimental to communities and the cause of death among children, particularly the under-fives, as well as pregnant women, women, and men in general. Preferably, readers may use the book as a bedside reference manual, especially those working in malaria endemic areas, which may contribute to reducing human suffering and unnecessary death. Although the treatment of different forms of malaria, ranging from uncomplicated to complicated malaria, is outlined, users of the book should go beyond bedside medicine to the communities and deal with the root cause of the problem, which is the mainstay of malaria control and prevention. These interventions can facilitate the wellbeing of the communities in the affected countries, thereby economic improvement and meaningful development may be achieved. And we can all jointly acknowledge and accept that "this is our problem" as opposed to "it is their problem." This therefore can help us deal with malaria as a communicable disease.

Fyson H. Kasenga, PhD, MPH
Deputy Vice Chancellor,
Malawi Adventist University,
Malamulo College of Health of Sciences,
Makwasa, Malawi

Chapter 1

Origin of Two Most Virulent Agents of Human Malaria: *Plasmodium falciparum* and *Plasmodium vivax*

Boundenga Larson

Abstract

Malaria is a protozoan disease caused by a parasite belonging to *Plasmodium* genus. Five species are known to infect humans: *Plasmodium falciparum, Plasmodium vivax, Plasmodium knowlesi, Plasmodium ovale, and Plasmodium malariae*. Among these species, *Plasmodium falciparum* and *Plasmodium vivax* account for more than 95% of all human malaria infections and thus pose a serious public health challenge. *Plasmodium falciparum* is highly prevalent in sub-Saharan Africa, while *Plasmodium vivax* is rare in sub-Saharan Africa but endemic in many parts of Asia. The recent studies using the development of molecular tools have shown that a large diversity of malaria parasites circulate among the nonhuman primates and certainly present a similarity with human parasites. For a long time, the question of the origin of its parasites that infect human population has been the subject of much debate. Today, it would seem that both most virulent agents of human malaria would come from African apes. Thus, this chapter tries to review available data about the origin of these two *Plasmodium* species.

Keywords: *Plasmodium*, nonhuman primate, human, Africa, origin, host switching

1. Introduction

Malaria is a serious infectious disease. It is caused by parasites of the genus *Plasmodium* and transmitted by *Anopheles* mosquitoes to its vertebrate hosts. This disease is an important global health problem, especially in sub-Saharan Africa [1] (**Figure 1**). Indeed, the African region continues to carry a disproportionately high share of the global malaria burden [1, 2]. Among five *Plasmodium* species which infect human, two species *Plasmodium falciparum* and *Plasmodium vivax* pose the greatest threat for human health. For example, *P. falciparum* is the most prevalent malaria parasite on the African continent. It is responsible for most malaria-related deaths globally [3], while *P. vivax* is rare in sub-Saharan Africa, but it is the major malaria parasite in most countries outside of sub-Saharan Africa [4].

The origin of parasites responsible of human malaria has always been at the center of the debate [5, 6]. Understanding the origin of its infectious agents could open a door in the improvement of strategies to fight against the malaria agents which constantly surprise us by their abilities to adapt to the different means of fight put in place. So then, the questions are as follows: *Where do the pathogens*

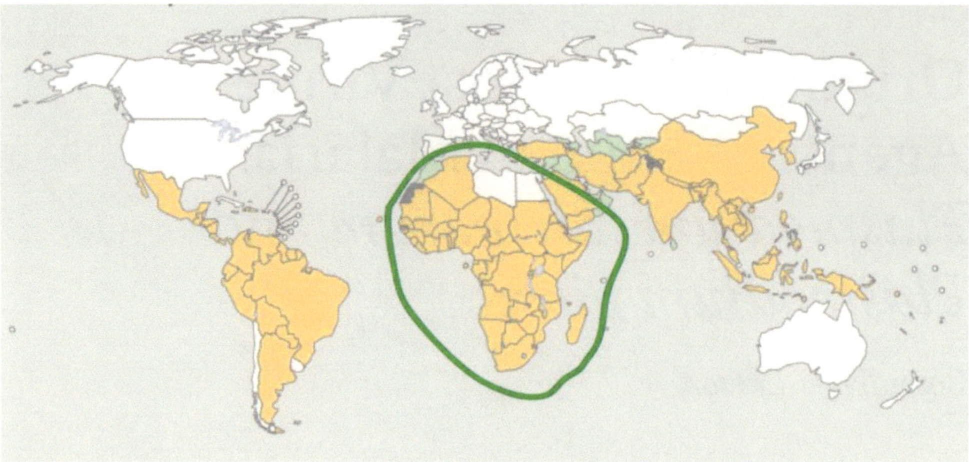

Figure 1.
Map of world malaria distribution.

responsible for this disease come from in humans? This chapter is a synthesis of the available data on the origin of two most virulent agents of human malaria: *P. falciparum* and *P. vivax*.

2. Nonhuman primate natural hosts of a large *Plasmodium* diversity

Today, the diversity of *Plasmodium* parasites infecting primates is well documented. First studies based in morphological analysis have reported three species which infect African apes (*Plasmodium reichenowi*, *Plasmodium schwetzi*, and *Plasmodium rodhaini*), and some of these were found to resemble human parasites *Plasmodium malariae*, *Plasmodium vivax*, and *Plasmodium ovale* [7]. The development of molecular tools allowed for a re-examination of *Plasmodium* diversity [8–10]. Data collected over the past years have shown that NHPs are infected with large diversity of *Plasmodium* belonging to two subgenera (*Laverania* and *Plasmodium*) [11] (**Figure 2**).

2.1 *Laverania* subgenus

Among species classified into *Laverania* group, four species infect chimpanzees (*P. gaboni*, *P. billcollinsi*, *P. billbrayi*, and *P. reichenowi*), only three infect gorillas (*P. adleri*, *P. blacklocki*, and *P. praefalciparum*), and only one infect bonobo (*P. lomamiensis*) [8, 9, 12]. Therefore, *P. billbrayi* [10] is not accepted as a new species by some authors [6, 13] who reported that these isolates did not seem to be sufficiently distinct from *P. gaboni* to warrant a separate species designation [6]. However, this species was described only in *Pan troglodytes schweinfurthii* and hence is the reason why we believe that could be another species [10] (**Figure 2**). Moreover, Mapua and colleagues reported recently several lineages of these parasites among African apes [14].

To date, all studies on natural populations of apes (based on the analysis of fecal samples) have shown that no *Plasmodium* species from the *Laverania* subgenus is able to infect *in natura* both hosts (gorillas and chimpanzees) [8, 13], thus suggesting the existence of a strong host specificity due to genetic barrier [6, 15]. However, a recent study revealed that this genetic barrier is not completely impermeable [16]; moreover, in this study, authors reported that the exchanges between gorillas

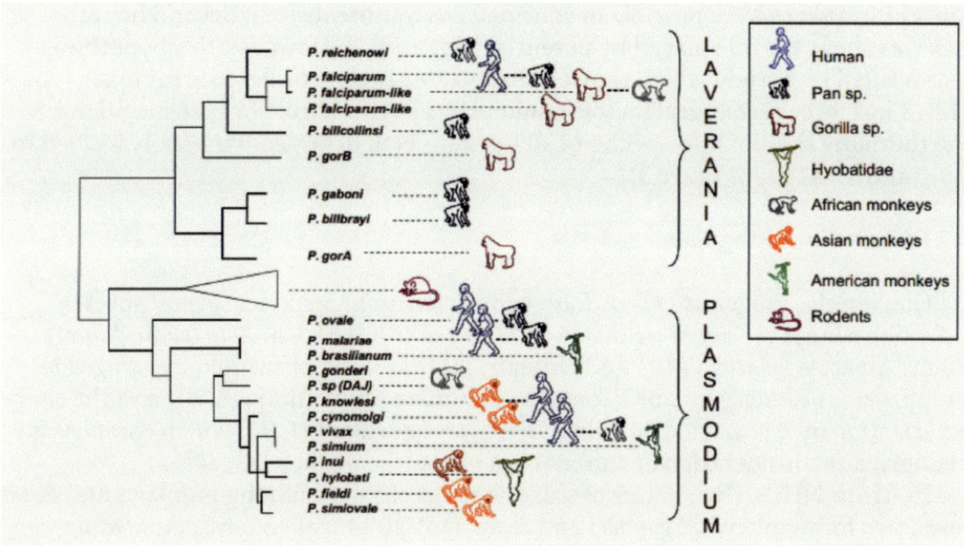

Figure 2.
The tree of relationship of primate Plasmodium with the currently known categories of hosts. Primate ***Plasmodium*** *is subdivided in two subgenera: Laverania and Plasmodium [11].*

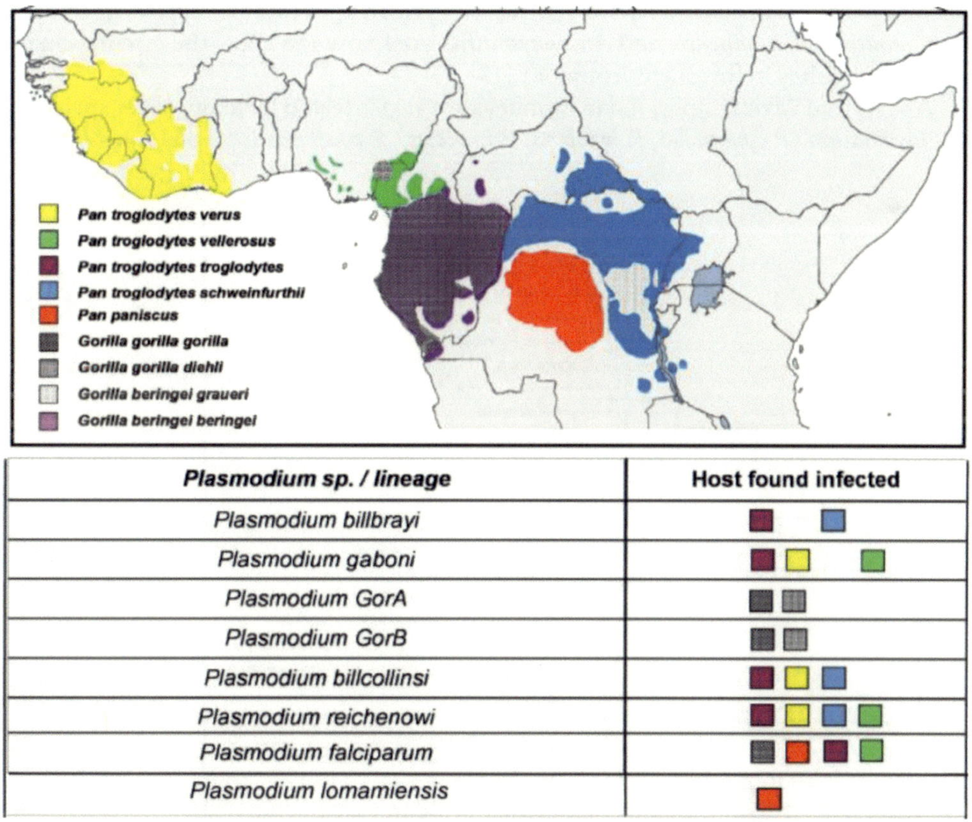

Figure 3.
Distribution of the different subspecies of great apes in Africa and representation of the spread of the different Plasmodium species in these species [5].

and chimpanzees were possible in confined environments [16]. Second hypothesis was about the role played by potential vectors [17]. However, this hypothesis was refuted by a study which showed that vectors had no preference for hosts [18]. Thus, other ecological factors could play a potential role in host specificity. Furthermore the simians' species of this group seem to be geographically located in central Africa only (**Figure 3**).

2.2 *Plasmodium* subgenus

Conversely, subgenus *Plasmodium* (non-*Laverania*) includes several species infecting a large variety of primates of varied origins [Africa, Asia (*catarrhines*), South America (*platyrrhines*) and Human] [11]. Two major facts concerning this group were the emergence of *P. knowlesi* in human population [19, 20] and the characterization of *P. vivax*-like in chimpanzees and gorillas [21, 22] which completely changed our consideration of this malaria parasite subgenus [23, 24].

In Africa NHPs, five species of this subgenus circulate among monkeys and great apes, two for monkeys (*P. gonderi* and *P.* sp. DAJ-2004 [called now *Plasmodium mandrilli* [25]]) and three for great apes (*P. vivax*-like, *P. malariae*-like, and *P. ovale*-like) [13, 16]. In African great apes, both hosts (chimpanzee and gorilla) are infected with these parasites (*P. vivax*-like, *P. malariae*-like, and *P. ovale*-like) (**Figures 3** and **4**). Thus, these *Plasmodium* species are not specific hosts, and it would be very interesting to establish the mechanisms which favor host switching for these parasites. Several species were reported as implicate in circulation of malaria parasites in central Africa [17, 18]. In African apes three *Anopheles* species (*An. moucheti*, *An. vinckei*, and *An. marshallii*) are known to allow the circulation of malaria parasites in forest environment [18].

Apart from African apes, Asian monkeys are also infected by many other species of *Plasmodium* (*P. cynomolgi*, *P. hylobati*, *P. knowlesi*, *P. coatneyi*, *P. fragile*, *P. fieldi*,

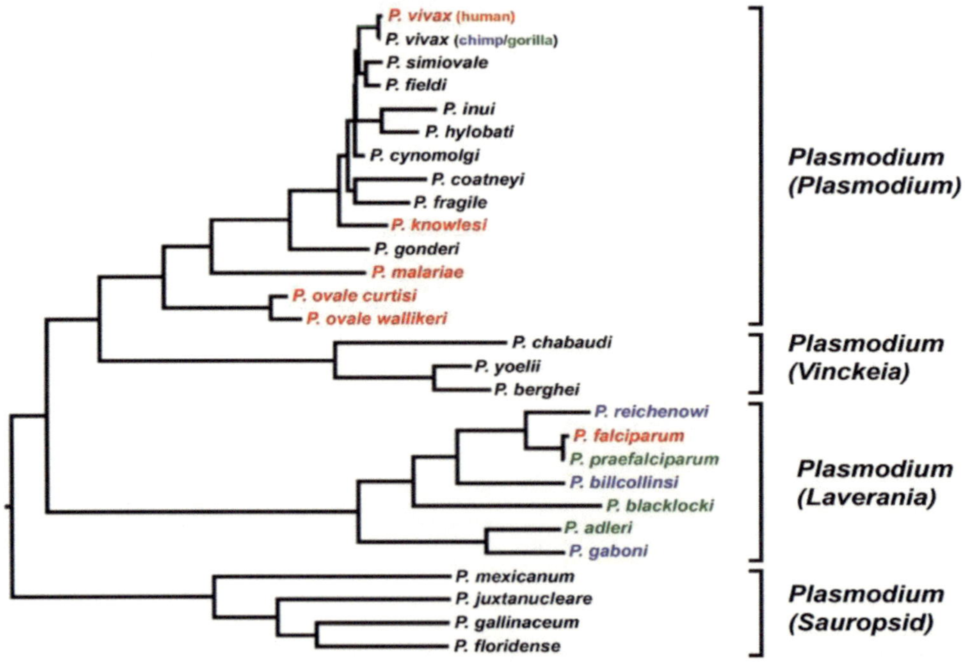

Figure 4.
Phylogenetic tree of some Plasmodium species found in apes.

P. simiovale, and *P inui Plasmodium* spp. [26]) (**Figures 3** and **4**). Several other species of *Plasmodium* were observed among Asian apes by microscopic analyses, but no molecular evidence of the existence of these lineages are available (e.g., *P. pithecia* and *P. sandoshami*). These malaria parasites could infect many apes' hosts. Several studies reported of the different NHP species with same parasites [27] or many parasites which were found in one species of NHP, for example, four species of simian malaria parasites were characterized in the pig-tailed macaques (*Macaca nemestrina*) [28, 29]. In this part of the world, the situation of *P. knowlesi* gives a good example of the risk that these parasites could present to humans. Recently, the probable existence of three divergent subpopulations of *P. knowlesi* with the different origins was reported [30].

Finally, in South America some *Plasmodium* species were described as infecting NHPs. The species found in Southern American primates are *Plasmodium brasilianum* and *Plasmodium simium*, and these parasite species naturally infect monkeys from the Cebidae and Atelidae families [31] (**Figure 3**). However, *P. brasilianum* infects 11 species of monkeys (*Alouatta spp*, *Ateles spp*, *Brachyteles arachnoides*, *Cacajao calvus*, *Callicebus spp*, *Cebus spp*, *Chiropotes satanas*, *Lagothrix spp*, *Saimiri spp*, *Saguinus midas*, and *Pithecia pithecia*), while *Plasmodium simium* infects only 2 species (*Alouatta spp* and *Brachyteles arachnoides*). In recent studies, *P. simium* was found for the first time in capuchin monkeys from the Brazilian Atlantic Forest [32]. *P. brasilium* and *P. simium* are similar and indistinguishable from human *P. malariae* and *P. vivax*. These similarities occur at the morphological, genetic, and immunological levels [31, 32].

3. Where do the malaria parasites that infect men come from?

The understanding of origin of human malaria parasites has been the subject of numerous studies that have been based on the morphology, biology, and affiliation of parasites to their hosts [33]. However, recent development of molecular tools in diagnosis has made considerable progress in understanding the evolutionary history of malaria parasites. Indeed, the contribution of several new sequences by this new approach will clarify the debate on many theories developed on the subject [34]. Moreover, several of these parasites have been found to be associated with humans by lateral transfer from other vertebrate host species [35, 36]. We will present the probable origin of two most virulent *Plasmodium* species that infect human.

3.1 *Plasmodium falciparum*

The debate on the origin of *P. falciparum* most spread in world (**Figure 5**) was opened with the study of Waters and his collaborators who proposed an avian origin of this parasite that is to say that the man would have recently acquired this parasite of a transfer from birds to humans [37]. Indeed, phylogenetic analyses based on the study of ribosomal RNA subunit (rRNA) sequences showed that *P. falciparum* formed a monophyletic group with *Plasmodium* spp. of birds (see **Figure 6**), hence the conclusion of the authors.

Three years after the first hypothesis on the origin of *P. falciparum*, Escalante and Ayala [38], in their study also based on 18S RNA, take into account for the first time *P. reichenowi*, an isolated parasite in a chimpanzee African (**Figure 7**). They will show that this parasite is the closest parent of *P. falciparum*; therefore, this observation allowed authors to conclude that *Plasmodium falciparum* origin was not a recent lateral transfer of this parasite of birds to humans [38, 39]. In this study, *P. falciparum* and *P. reichenowi* form a large group with primate parasites of the subgenus *Plasmodium* (*non-Laverania*), rodents, and birds [38, 40, 41] (**Figure 7**). This will further fuel the debate on the origin of *P. falciparum*.

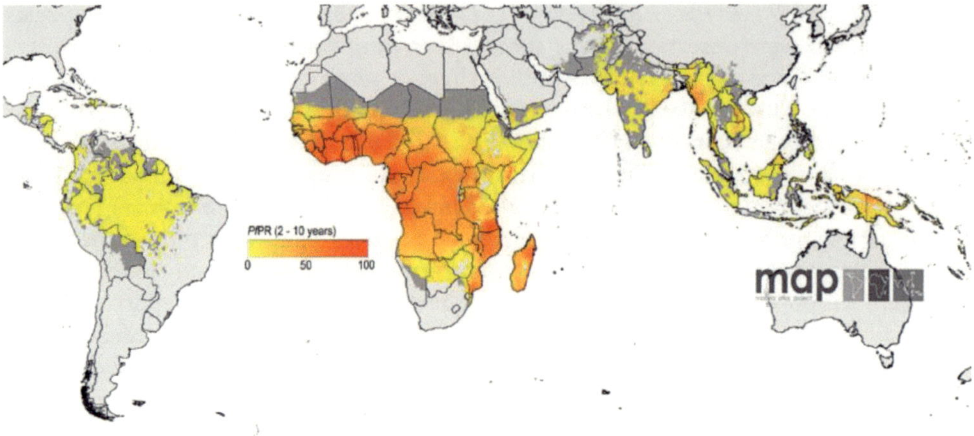

Figure 5.
Distribution of Plasmodium falciparum in the world [42].

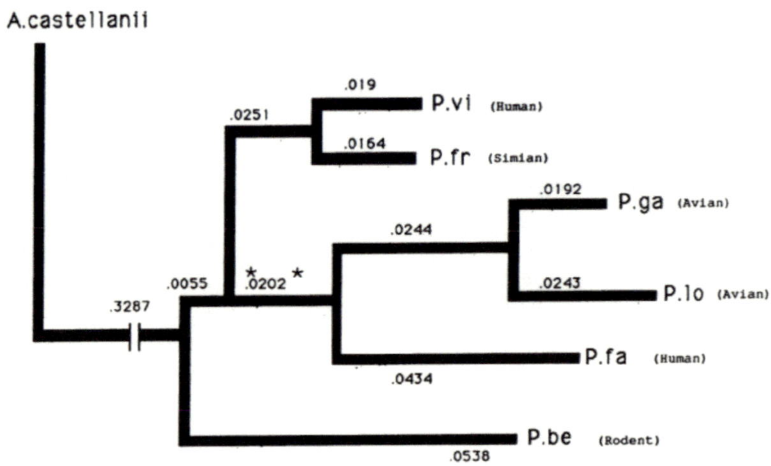

Figure 6.
Phylogenetic tree of malaria parasites obtained by Waters and colleagues [37].

The disputes surround the probable origin of *P. falciparum*, whether it comes from birds or rodents, will be raging. Authors as Prugnolle et al. believe that the problems or weaknesses of many studies were based essentially on two aspects [5]: firstly the low number of plasmodial species and sequences integrated in these analyses and secondly the limited number of molecular markers used for the development of phylogenies. Despite all this controversy, *P. falciparum* will be considered to have an African origin [43–45].

The year 2009 will completely change our understanding of the evolutionary history of *P. falciparum*, because prior to this year, only one species (*P. reichenowi*) was known to be closer to *P. falciparum*. After the discovery of *Plasmodium gaboni* parasite that infects chimpanzees [46], several other sequences from African great apes will definitively bring elements of answers to question on the origin of this parasite.

Indeed, in 2010, Prugnolle and colleagues will highlight for the first time *P. falciparum*-like in gorillas and several other lineages. These studies will prove that the *Laverania* group that includes *P. falciparum* has a great diversity of species that circulate in African primates [9]. This will make it possible to show that the origin

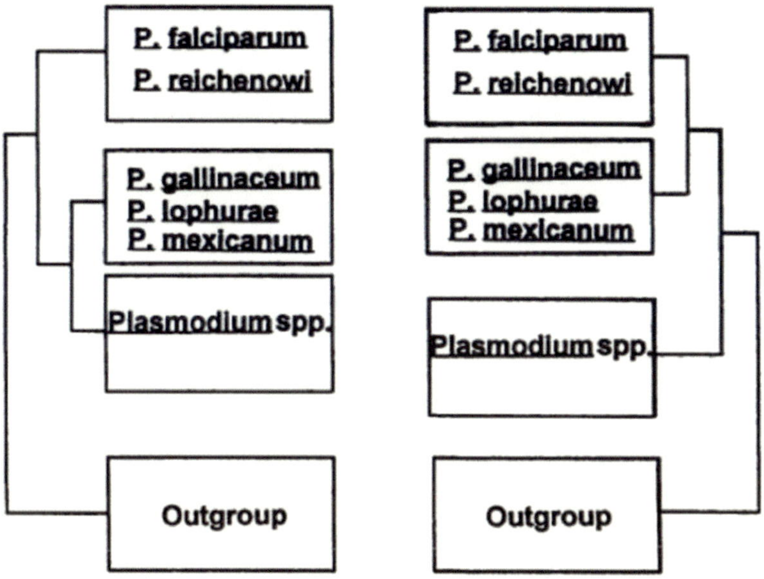

Figure 7.
Two ML phylogenetic trees obtained by grouping 11 Plasmodium species as indicated (the six unlisted species are grouped as Plasmodium spp.) [38].

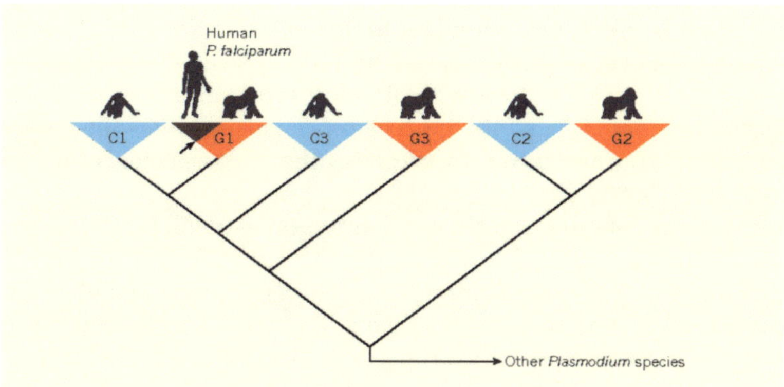

Figure 8.
Origin of human Plasmodium falciparum. This phylogenetic tree illustrates the remarkable diversity of Plasmodium parasites infecting African apes (Holmes 2010).

of *P. falciparum* is not found in birds or rodents but in the gorillas that have recently transmitted it to humans via anophobic zoo-anthropophilic mosquito [17, 18]. *P. falciparum*-like of gorillas will be named *P. praefalciparum* to distinguish it from that which infects humans [11, 13].

In 2011, the hypothesis of a gorilla origin of *P. falciparum* seems to be weakened by the discovery of *P. praefalciparum* in a small African monkey (*Cercopithecus nictitans*) [47]. This study also will reveal the existence of at least two types of *P. praefalciparum*: 1 and 2. *P. praefalciparum*-1 infects gorillas and monkeys (*C. nictitans*), and *P. praefalciparum*-2 infects only gorillas [11]. Other studies will focus on African monkeys, but will not find *P. praefalciparum* [48]. Thus, we believe that the hypothesis of *Plasmodium falciparum* from monkeys is not solid and that *C. nictitans* species is not a natural reservoir for this parasite [48].

Today, after numerous studies that analyzed more than 5000 samples of wild and captives apes [8–10, 12, 13, 16, 21, 22, 47] (**Figure 8**), it appears that gorillas are the reservoir for the *P. praefalciparum*, even though several hypotheses concerning the origin of *P. falciparum* have been proposed for primates [10, 47].

The hypothesis according to which *Plasmodium falciparum* would come from gorillas seems to be the most plausible at the moment. Indeed, several *P. praefalciparum* sequences had been found from numerous wild-living gorillas in different areas [8, 13]. Loy and colleagues suggested that this parasite strain that was able to cross the host species barrier by carried one or more highly unusual mutations that conferred him an ability to colonize humans [49]. This theory comes to the fact that recent studies in human populations living close to the wild apes did not reveal the presence of parasites of great apes belonging to *Laverania* subgenus in humans [50, 51]. Thus, then it would seem that *P. falciparum* comes from African gorillas according to available data at the moment.

3.2 Origin of *Plasmodium vivax*

Plasmodium vivax is particularly prevalent in Asia, Southeast Asia, South America, and the Western Pacific region [52] (**Figure 9**). Already the first studies on malaria of the great apes had revealed the presence of parasites resembling *P. vivax* [53, 54]. Despite its first observations, the question on the origin of *P. vivax* remained uncertain for several years. Concerning this interesting question of the *P. vivax* origin, several hypotheses have been proposed in recent years.

The first hypotheses about the origin of *P. vivax* had suggested that it originated in Southeast Asia [24, 49]. These hypotheses were based on the fact that *P. vivax* shares morphological and biological traits with several macaque parasites and that *Plasmodium* simian's species are abundant in this Asian region [36]. This hypothesis was supported by the phylogenetic analyses that placed *P. vivax* among the *Plasmodium* spp. of Asian monkeys with like closest parent, *Plasmodium cynomolgi*, which infects macaques in Asia [40, 55]. The consensus view has thus been that *P. vivax* emerged in southeastern Asia following the cross-species transmission of a macaque parasite [23, 56, 57].

In addition to the first hypothesis, another hypothesis will articulate around of the negative Duffy receptor and would suggest African origin of *P. vivax* [58, 59]. Indeed, the presence of negative Duffy blood group in central and West African populations was correlated with the absence of *P. vivax*. This character would confer resistance to *P. vivax* infection, which suggested that this mutation arose in response to prolonged selection pressure from *P. vivax* [60]. Currently, Duffy antigen is the

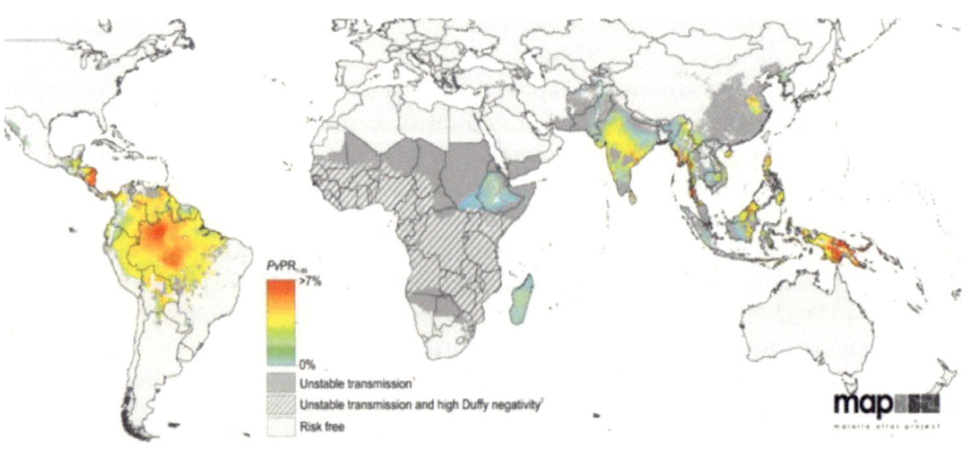

Figure 9.
The spatial distribution of Plasmodium vivax in the world [52].

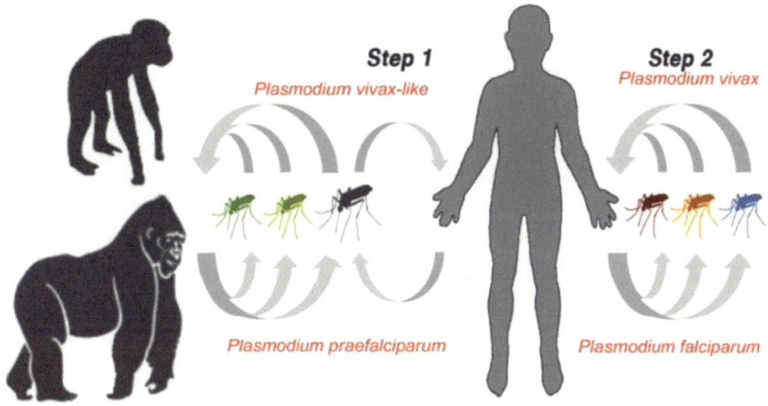

Figure 10.
The diagram presents a possible two-step scenario for the transfer and establishment of ape malarias in humans. Sylvatic anopheline vectors were transmitting malaria between apes; in the first step, one (or more) bridge vector(s) would also transfer infective Plasmodium parasites to humans. In a second step, human-adapted Plasmodium parasites adapted to domesticated mosquito vector species that share the same ecological niche with humans [63].

only receptor known to be used by parasite to invade the red blood cell. Thus, it has been proposed that *P. vivax* co-evolved with African populations for longer than with other human populations [24, 61].

However, the recent studies using the development of molecular tools allow to have a clear view on the origin of this parasite. These studies have shown that chimpanzees and gorillas from central and West Africa harbor a large diversity of *P. vivax*-like parasites [10, 21, 22, 62]. This discovery accentuates the African origin of *Plasmodium vivax* and reveals that African great apes are potential sylvatic reservoir of *P. vivax* [21, 22]. However, elucidation of the origin of *P. vivax* in African apes needed complementary studies of wild-living populations across central Africa [22].

Also, Prugnolle et al. have shown that *P. vivax*-like found among African great apes form a distinct and much more diverse genetic group than that of human parasites [21]. In this study authors revealed also an older origin of the African simian lineages and the fact that these lineages are able to infect the Caucasian population today [21] (**Figure 10**). Thus, the discovery of *P. vivax* in large numbers of chimpanzees and gorillas provides compelling evidence for an African, rather than an Asian, origin of human *P. vivax*.

Today, an interesting question would be to understand how this passage of apes to man had been done. To this question, in view of current data and analyses, we agree to say, instead, it is much more likely that extant human *P. vivax* could represent a lineage that survived after spreading out of Africa [21, 64, 65], because this theory could explain the fact that we observed today a reduced diversity of the human parasites which would result from an out-of-Africa bottleneck, such as observed in *P. falciparum* [45, 66].

4. Malaria like a zoonotic disease: the running toward new environments is a wont for *Plasmodium*

It is true that many *Plasmodium* parasites circulating in African NHPs could produce symptoms of this disease in apes [67]. However, no *Plasmodium* species particularly parasites belonging to *Laverania* subgenus has been found to infect human to date. Studies conducted in rural population in central Africa (Cameroon and Gabon) have shown that *Laverania* parasites were absent of human populations living in villages that are in very close proximity to wild forest [50, 51] and even those working in very close contact with NHPs [16]. On the other hand, several studies reported that *P. falciparum* is able to infect African apes, for example, Bonobos, chimpanzees [10, 26], and recently the mandrills [16]. The question is *why these transfers are rare or why the ancestral parent of P. falciparum (P. praefalciparum) appear incapable of infecting humans today*. Loy et al. suggest that gorilla parasite strain that was able to cross the host species barrier must have carried one or more highly unusual mutations that enable it to colonize humans [49]. But, supplementary studies would be necessary to support this hypothesis.

In contrast, many parasites of *Plasmodium* subgenus were reported to infect humans. The major case known is *P. knowlesi* that infects NHPs in south Asia and now is considered as the fifth *Plasmodium* species that infects human and cause malaria in southern Asian population [19]. Other cases of natural or accidental infections of humans with simians *Plasmodium* were reported in literature. Indeed, a total of seven species of monkey malaria have been reported via mosquitoes (*P. cynomolgi*, *P. brasilianum*, *P. eylesi*, *P. knowlesi*, *P. inui*, *P. schwetzi*, and *P. simium*) [11, 68, 69]. Recently, ape *P. vivax* has been found to cause clinical malaria in Caucasians who stayed during some days in African forest [21]. Thus, parasites of *Plasmodium* subgenus are apparently able to cross the species barrier to humans. So the emergence of these parasites should be monitored in areas where an influx of contact between humans and NHPs increases with anthropization, which destroys ape habitat and favors contact. In view of the rare faction of monkeys and the increase of the human population, it is feared that human infection of simians *Plasmodium* will become more frequent which could lead to humans becoming simians' major host [70].

5. Prevention

The potential for zoonosis is influenced by human habitation and behavior as well as the adaptive capabilities of parasites and vectors. Indeed, the existence of potential sylvatic reservoirs of *P. vivax* and *P. falciparum* in Africa could compromise malaria control and eradication efforts. Actually, there is lack of knowledge about the real extent of malaria zoonosis. Thus, this aspect of zoonosis malaria parasites must be taken into account by the public health authorities responsible for the fight against malaria. African structures health need to put appropriate strategies of prevention against zoonotic malaria parasites that could be developed. However, they must be based on good data of research on diagnosis and treatment of zoonotic malaria. Moreover, all people living in the locality or monkeys are known to grass a large variety of malaria parasite, which must take their precaution when they venture into forest environment, in order to avoid mosquito bites.

6. Conclusion

The development of the tools of molecular biology allowed us to see clearer in the history of parasite that infects the man, especially *Plasmodium* species. Indeed, these tools allowed us to highlight large diversity of the malaria parasites that circulate to the nonhuman primates, so to understand better the origin of the most virulent parasite responsible for human malaria (*Plasmodium falciparum* and *Plasmodium vivax*). Therefore, on the basis of available data, it is more than likely that its parasites have an African origin and that African gorillas and chimpanzees would constitute potential reservoirs of its parasites. Thus, in this context, it is important to determine or develop appropriate preventive strategies. It is necessary to set up monitoring systems in forest areas and to make sensitization campaigns.

Annex for reader

Diversity: the condition of having or being composed of differing elements (variety). It can also include of different species or genetic lineages.

Gorilla sp.: designs all species belonging to *Gorilla* genus. This genus has three subspecies of *gorilla* (*Gorilla gorilla gorilla; Gorilla gorilla graueri* and *Gorilla gorilla beringei*).

Laverania: is a subgenus of the *Plasmodium* genus of parasites. The parasites belonging to this subgenus have a strong host specificity.

Outgroup: outgroup is a more distantly related group of organisms that serves as a reference group when determining the evolutionary relationships of the ingroup, and it is used as a point of comparison for the ingroup and specifically allows for the phylogeny to be rooted.

Phylogenetic tree: a phylogenetic tree is a diagram that represents evolutionary relationships among organisms.

Plasmodium GorA (Prugnolle et al. 2010): *Plasmodium adleri.*

Plasmodium gorB (Prugnolle et al. 2010): *Plasmodium blacklocki.*

Plasmodium (non-*Laverania*): non-Laverania subgenus includes many parasites such as *P. malariae*, *P. vivax*, *P. ovale-curtisi*, and *P. ovale-wallikeri* as well as the monkey parasites *P. inui* and *P. hylobati*.

Pan sp.: *Pan* sp. designs all species belonging to *Pan* genus (the common name of member of this genus chimpanzees and bonobo).

RNA subunit (rRNA): ribosomal ribonucleic acid (rRNA) is the RNA component of the ribosome and is an essential element for protein synthesis in all living organisms.

Author details

Boundenga Larson
Centre International de Recherches Médicales de Franceville (CIRMF), Franceville, Gabon

*Address all correspondence to: boundenga@gmail.com

References

[1] WHO. Malaria Rapid Diagnostic Test Performance: Summary Results of WHO Product Testing of Malaria RDTs: Round 1-8 (2008-2018). 2018

[2] WHO. Malaria Rapid Diagnostic Test Performance: Results of WHO Product Testing of Malaria RDTs: Round 7 (2016-2017). 2017

[3] Bhatt S, Weiss DJ, Cameron E, Bisanzio D, Mappin B, Dalrymple U, et al. The effect of malaria control on *Plasmodium falciparum* in Africa between 2000 and 2015. Nature. 2015;**526**:207-211

[4] WHO. World Malaria Report 2014. World Health Organization; 2015

[5] Prugnolle F, Durand P, Ollomo B, Duval L, Ariey F, Arnathau C, et al. A fresh look at the origin of *Plasmodium falciparum*, the most malignant malaria agent. PLoS Pathogens. 2011;7:e1001283

[6] Rayner JC, Liu W, Peeters M, Sharp PM, Hahn BH. A plethora of *Plasmodium* species in wild apes: A source of human infection? Trends in Parasitology. 2011;**27**:222-229

[7] Snounou G, Escalante A, Kasenene J, Rénia L, Grüner AC, Krief S. Le paludisme chez les hominides. Bulletin de l'Académie Nationale de Médecine. 2011;**195**:1945-1954

[8] Boundenga L, Ollomo B, Rougeron V, Mouele LY, Mve-Ondo B, Delicat-Loembet LM, et al. Diversity of malaria parasites in great apes in Gabon. Malaria Journal. 2015;**14**:111

[9] Prugnolle F, Durand P, Neel C, Ollomo B, Ayala FJ, Arnathau C, et al. African great apes are natural hosts of multiple related malaria species, including *Plasmodium falciparum*. Proceedings of the National Academy of Sciences of the United States of America. 2010;**107**:1458-1463

[10] Krief S, Escalante AA, Pacheco MA, Mugisha L, Andre C, Halbwax M, et al. On the diversity of malaria parasites in African apes and the origin of *Plasmodium falciparum* from bonobos. PLoS Pathogens. 2010;**6**:e1000765

[11] Gonzalez JP, Prugnolle F, Leroy E. Men, primates, and germs: An ongoing affair. Current Topics in Microbiology and Immunology. 2013;**365**:337-353

[12] Liu W, Sherrill-Mix S, Learn GH, Scully EJ, Li Y, Avitto AN, et al. Wild bonobos host geographically restricted malaria parasites including a putative new Laverania species. Nature Communications. 2017;**8**:1635

[13] Liu W, Li Y, Learn GH, Rudicell RS, Robertson JD, Keele BF, et al. Origin of the human malaria parasite *Plasmodium falciparum* in gorillas. Nature. 2010;**467**:420-425

[14] Mapua MI, Petrzelkova KJ, Burgunder J, Dadakova E, Brozova K, Hrazdilova K, et al. A comparative molecular survey of malaria prevalence among eastern chimpanzee populations in Issa Valley (Tanzania) and Kalinzu (Uganda). Malaria Journal. 2016;**15**:423

[15] Forni D, Pontremoli C, Cagliani R, Pozzoli U, Clerici M, Sironi M. Positive selection underlies the species-specific binding of *Plasmodium falciparum* RH5 to human basigin. Molecular Ecology. 2015;**24**:4711-4722

[16] Ngoubangoye B, Boundenga L, Arnathau C, Mombo IM, Durand P, Tsoumbou TA, et al. The host specificity of ape malaria parasites can be broken in confined environments. International Journal for Parasitology. 2016;**46**:737-744

[17] Paupy C, Makanga B, Ollomo B, Rahola N, Durand P, Magnus J, et al. Anopheles moucheti and Anopheles vinckei are candidate vectors of ape *Plasmodium* parasites, including *Plasmodium praefalciparum* in Gabon. PLoS One. 2013;**8**:e57294

[18] Makanga B, Yangari P, Rahola N, Rougeron V, Elguero E, Boundenga L, et al. Ape malaria transmission and potential for ape-to-human transfers in Africa. Proceedings of the National Academy of Sciences of the United States of America. 2016;**113**:5329-5334

[19] Cox-Singh J, Singh B. Knowlesi malaria: Newly emergent and of public health importance? Trends in Parasitology. 2008;**24**:406-410

[20] White NJ. *Plasmodium knowlesi*: The fifth human malaria parasite. Clinical Infectious Diseases. 2008;**46**:172-173

[21] Prugnolle F, Rougeron V, Becquart P, Berry A, Makanga B, Rahola N, et al. Diversity, host switching and evolution of *Plasmodium vivax* infecting African great apes. Proceedings of the National Academy of Sciences of the United States of America. 2013;**110**:8123-8128

[22] Liu W, Li Y, Shaw KS, Learn GH, Plenderleith LJ, Malenke JA, et al. African origin of the malaria parasite *Plasmodium vivax*. Nature Communications. 2014;**5**:3346

[23] Mu J, Joy DA, Duan J, Huang Y, Carlton J, Walker J, et al. Host switch leads to emergence of *Plasmodium vivax* malaria in humans. Molecular Biology and Evolution. 2005;**22**:1686-1693

[24] Cornejo OE, Escalante AA. The origin and age of *Plasmodium vivax*. Trends in Parasitology. 2006;**22**:558-563

[25] Boundenga L, Ngoubangoye B, Mombo IM, Tsoubmou TA, Renaud F, Rougeron V, et al. Extensive diversity of malaria parasites circulating in central African bats and monkeys. Ecology and Evolution. 2018;**8**:10578-10586

[26] Pacheco MA, Cranfield M, Cameron K, Escalante AA. Malarial parasite diversity in chimpanzees: The value of comparative approaches to ascertain the evolution of *Plasmodium falciparum* antigens. Malaria Journal. 2013;**12**:328

[27] Divis PC, Singh B, Anderios F, Hisam S, Matusop A, Kocken CH, et al. Admixture in humans of two divergent *Plasmodium knowlesi* populations associated with different macaque host species. PLoS Pathogens. 2015;**11**:e1004888

[28] Eyles DE, Fong YL, Warren M, Guinn E, Sandosham A, Wharton R. *Plasmodium coatneyi*, a new species of primate malaria from Malaya. The American Journal of Tropical Medicine and Hygiene. 1962;**11**:597-604

[29] Vythilingam I, Hii J. Simian malaria parasites: Special emphasis on *Plasmodium knowlesi* and their Anopheles vectors in Southeast Asia. In: Anopheles Mosquitoes-New Insights into Malaria Vectors. Rijeka: InTech; 2013

[30] Divis PC, Lin LC, Rovie-Ryan JJ, Kadir KA, Anderios F, Hisam S, et al. Three divergent subpopulations of the malaria parasite *Plasmodium knowlesi*. Emerging Infectious Diseases. 2017;**23**:616-624

[31] de Castro Duarte AMR, dos Santos Malafronte R, Cerutti C Jr, Curado I, de Paiva BR, Maeda AY, et al. Natural Plasmodium infections in Brazilian wild monkeys: Reservoirs for human infections? Acta Tropica. 2008;**107**:179-185

[32] de Alvarenga DA, de Pina-Costa A, de Sousa TN, Pissinatti A, Zalis MG, Suarez-Mutis MC, et al. Simian malaria in the Brazilian Atlantic forest: First description of natural infection of

capuchin monkeys (Cebinae subfamily) by *Plasmodium simium*. Malaria Journal. 2015;**14**:81

[33] Cserti CM, Dzik WH. The ABO blood group system and *Plasmodium falciparum* malaria. Blood. 2007;**110**:2250-2258

[34] Das A, Bajaj R, Mohanty S, Swain V. Genetic diversity and evolutionary history of *Plasmodium falciparum* and *P. vivax*. Current Science. 2007:1516-1524

[35] Garnham P. Immunity against the different stages of malaria parasites. Bulletin de la Societe de pathologie exotique et de ses filiales. 1966;**59**:549-557

[36] Garnham PCC. Malaria Parasites and Other Haemosporidia. Oxford, England: Blackwell; Philadelphia: Davis; 1966. 1132 pp

[37] Waters A, Higgins D, McCutchan T. *Plasmodium falciparum* appears to have arisen as a result of lateral transfer between avian and human hosts. Proceedings of the National Academy of Sciences. 1991;**88**:3140-3144

[38] Escalante AA, Ayala FJ. Phylogeny of the malarial genus *Plasmodium*, derived from rRNA gene sequences. Proceedings of the National Academy of Sciences. 1994;**91**:11373-11377

[39] Escalante AA, Ayala FJ. Evolutionary origin of *Plasmodium* and other Apicomplexa based on rRNA genes. Proceedings of the National Academy of Sciences. 1995;**92**:5793-5797

[40] Perkins SL, Schall J. A molecular phylogeny of malarial parasites recovered from cytochrome b gene sequences. Journal of Parasitology. 2002;**88**:972-978

[41] Escalante AA, Lal AA, Ayala FJ. Genetic polymorphism and natural selection in the malaria parasite *Plasmodium falciparum*. Genetics. 1998;**149**:189-202

[42] Hay SI, Guerra CA, Gething PW, Patil AP, Tatem AJ, Noor AM, et al. A World Malaria Map: Plasmodium falciparum Endemicity in 2007. https://doi.org/10.1371/journal.pmed.1000048

[43] Pearce-Duvet JM. The origin of human pathogens: Evaluating the role of agriculture and domestic animals in the evolution of human disease. Biological Reviews of the Cambridge Philosophical Society. 2006;**81**:369-382

[44] Joy DA, Feng X, Mu J, Furuya T, Chotivanich K, Krettli AU, et al. Early origin and recent expansion of *Plasmodium falciparum*. Science. 2003;**300**:318-321

[45] Conway DJ, Fanello C, Lloyd JM, Al-Joubori BM, Baloch AH, Somanath SD, et al. Origin of *Plasmodium falciparum* malaria is traced by mitochondrial DNA. Molecular and Biochemical Parasitology. 2000;**111**:163-171

[46] Ollomo B, Durand P, Prugnolle F, Douzery E, Arnathau C, Nkoghe D, et al. A new malaria agent in African hominids. PLoS Pathogens. 2009;**5**:e1000446

[47] Prugnolle F, Ollomo B, Durand P, Yalcindag E, Arnathau C, Elguero E, et al. African monkeys are infected by *Plasmodium falciparum* nonhuman primate-specific strains. Proceedings of the National Academy of Sciences of the United States of America. 2011;**108**:11948-11953

[48] Ayouba A, Mouacha F, Learn GH, Mpoudi-Ngole E, Rayner JC, Sharp PM, et al. Ubiquitous Hepatocystis infections, but no evidence of *Plasmodium falciparum*-like malaria parasites in wild greater spot-nosed monkeys (*Cercopithecus nictitans*). International Journal for Parasitology. 2012;**42**:709-713

[49] Loy DE, Liu W, Li Y, Learn GH, Plenderleith LJ, Sundararaman SA, et al. Out of Africa: Origins and evolution of the human malaria parasites *Plasmodium falciparum* and *Plasmodium vivax*. International Journal for Parasitology. 2017;**47**:87-97

[50] Delicat-Loembet L, Rougeron V, Ollomo B, Arnathau C, Roche B, Elguero E, et al. No evidence for ape *Plasmodium* infections in humans in Gabon. PLoS One. 2015;**10**:e0126933

[51] Sundararaman SA, Liu W, Keele BF, Learn GH, Bittinger K, Mouacha F, et al. *Plasmodium falciparum*-like parasites infecting wild apes in southern Cameroon do not represent a recurrent source of human malaria. Proceedings of the National Academy of Sciences of the United States of America. 2013;**110**:7020-7025

[52] Allgower A, Taylor WR, Chappuis F, Eperon G. *Plasmodium vivax*, un parasite qui sort de l'ombre: *Plasmodium vivax*, a parasite coming out of the shadows. Revue Médicale Suisse. 2016;**12**:876-881

[53] Duval L, Fourment M, Nerrienet E, Rousset D, Sadeuh SA, Goodman SM, et al. African apes as reservoirs of *Plasmodium falciparum* and the origin and diversification of the *Laverania subgenus*. Proceedings of the National Academy of Sciences of the United States of America. 2010;**107**:10561-10566

[54] Duval L, Nerrienet E, Rousset D, Sadeuh Mba SA, Houze S, Fourment M, et al. Chimpanzee malaria parasites related to *Plasmodium ovale* in Africa. PLoS One. 2009;**4**:e5520

[55] Tachibana S-I, Sullivan SA, Kawai S, Nakamura S, Kim HR, Goto N, et al. *Plasmodium cynomolgi* genome sequences provide insight into *Plasmodium vivax* and the monkey malaria clade. Nature Genetics. 2012;**44**:1051

[56] Escalante AA, Cornejo OE, Freeland DE, Poe AC, Durrego E, Collins WE, et al. A monkey's tale: The origin of *Plasmodium vivax* as a human malaria parasite. Proceedings of the National Academy of Sciences. 2005;**102**:1980-1985

[57] Neafsey DE, Galinsky K, Jiang RH, Young L, Sykes SM, Saif S, et al. The malaria parasite *Plasmodium vivax* exhibits greater genetic diversity than *Plasmodium falciparum*. Nature Genetics. 2012;**44**:1046

[58] Culleton R, Carter R. African *Plasmodium vivax*: Distribution and origins. International Journal for Parasitology. 2012;**42**:1091-1097

[59] Livingstone FB. The Duffy blood groups, vivax malaria, and malaria selection in human populations: A review. Human Biology;**1984**:413-425

[60] Miller LH, Mason SJ, Clyde DF, McGinniss MH. The resistance factor to *Plasmodium vivax* in blacks: The Duffy-blood-group genotype, FyFy. New England Journal of Medicine. 1976;**295**:302-304

[61] Carter R, Mendis KN. Evolutionary and historical aspects of the burden of malaria. Clinical Microbiology Reviews. 2002;**15**:564-594

[62] Kaiser M, Lowa A, Ulrich M, Ellerbrok H, Goffe AS, Blasse A, et al. Wild chimpanzees infected with 5 *Plasmodium* species. Emerging Infectious Diseases. 2010;**16**:1956-1959

[63] Molina-Cruz A, Barillas-Mury C. Mosquito vectors of ape malarias: Another piece of the puzzle. Proceedings of the National Academy of Sciences of the United States of America. 2016;**113**:5153-5154

[64] Gilabert A, Otto TD, Rutledge GG, Franzon B, Ollomo B, Arnathau C, et al. *Plasmodium vivax*-like

genome sequences shed new insights into *Plasmodium vivax* biology and evolution. PLoS Biology. 2018;**16**:e2006035

[65] Loy DE, Plenderleith LJ, Sundararaman SA, Liu W, Gruszczyk J, Chen YJ, et al. Evolutionary history of human *Plasmodium vivax* revealed by genome-wide analyses of related ape parasites. Proceedings of the National Academy of Sciences of the United States of America. 2018;**115**:E8450-e8459

[66] Tanabe K, Mita T, Jombart T, Eriksson A, Horibe S, Palacpac N, et al. *Plasmodium falciparum* accompanied the human expansion out of Africa. Current Biology. 2010;**20**:1283-1289

[67] Herbert A, Boundenga L, Meyer A, Moukodoum DN, Okouga AP, Arnathau C, et al. Malaria-like symptoms associated with a natural *Plasmodium reichenowi* infection in a chimpanzee. Malaria Journal. 2015;**14**:220

[68] Ta TH, Hisam S, Lanza M, Jiram AI, Ismail N, Rubio JM. First case of a naturally acquired human infection with *Plasmodium cynomolgi*. Malaria Journal. 2014;**13**:68

[69] Lalremruata A, Magris M, Vivas-Martínez S, Koehler M, Esen M, Kempaiah P, et al. Natural infection of *Plasmodium brasilianum* in humans: Man and monkey share quartan malaria parasites in the Venezuelan Amazon. eBioMedicine. 2015;**2**:1186-1192

[70] Rodhain F. Is malaria a zoonotic infection? Bulletin de l'Académie Vétérinaire de France. 2012;**165**:335-338

Chapter 2

Malarial Pathophysiology and Phytochemical Interventions: A Current Discourse on Oxidative Stress Anti-Disease Phytotherapeutics

Greanious Alfred Mavondo, Blessing Nkazimulo Mkhwanazi, Joy Mavondo, Wisdom Peresuh and Obadiah Moyo

Abstract

Malarial systemic pathophysiology refers to physiological changes or abnormalities that are experienced by individuals infected with the *Plasmodium* parasite not be presenting in the absence of active, chronic or previous infection. The pathologies are derived, in part, from OS induced insults whose mediators are readily available in malaria. The malaria disease is equivalent to the pathophysiology as shown by the abnormal syndromic expressions ranging from ailments that affect homeostatic mechanisms and processes to tissues and organ specific damages and derangements. Phytotherapeutic remedies refer to the natural phytochemicals or plant medicinal compounds and their derivatives with known antiparasitic and antimalarial disease effects in both experimental and clinical situations. The chapter explores how *Plasmodium* infection generates or cause to be generated oxidative stress, how oxidative stress drives systemic disease process and how phytotherapeutics treatment (artemisinins) and administration (asiatic acid) in malaria resolves the various pathologies as a current situational analysis.

Keywords: malaria, phytochemicals, phytotherapeutics, asiatic acid, artemisinin, severe malaria anemia, *Plasmodium falciparum*, oxidative stress, reactive oxygen species, anti-disease

1. Introduction

Inferences into free radicals' release and their subsequent OS generation has been described as the causes and drivers of malaria [1–3]. The *Plasmodium* [4]-free radical production [5]-antioxidant defense systems [6] triumvirate axis may be elaborate in the host cell as a pathologic apparatus triggered to subside malarial infection intensity. The character of OS has scarcer shades of clarity up to date with some authors insinuating a protective facilitation against malaria disease, others claim a pathophysiologic role in the pathogenesis of the disease [6]. Studies, however, tend to associate the production of reactive oxygen (ROS) and nitrogenous species (RNS) with OS (OS) in the development of complex sequalae and systemic malarial disease and its outcomes.

Malarial parasite infection invokes hydroxyl free radical ($OH^{\cdot}$) production by the hepatocytes which may induce OS and apoptosis of liver parenchymal cells [7]. Additionally, it has been observed that parasitized red blood cells (pRBCs) generate $OH^{\cdot}$ radicals and H_2O_2 at approximately double the concentration found in non-parasitized red blood cells (npRBCs); an elicitation from the abundant intracell and endogenous redox reaction players.

Free hemoglobin (Hb), copiously available in malaria, is also a readily obtainable foundation of free radicals as the *Plasmodium* parasite uses the Fe^{2+}-containing molecule as a fountain of amino acids crucial for its sustenance during the erythrocytic stage of disease. The main component and source of protein-bound and free Fe^{2+} is high levels of haeme. The haeme-Fe^{2+} complex induces intravascular OS with deleterious conformational changes to the red blood cells (RBC's) and the endothelial cells. Consequentially, release from pRBC's during haemolysis and subsequent internalization of malarial parasites into liver and brain tissues ensues with varied malarial syndromes presentations [8].

Generally, free haem release during cell haemolysis has a prospective capacity of increasing OS through the Fenton-Fritz Haber-Joseph Joshua Weiss reaction [9, 10] which iron catalyzes, mainly: $Fe^{3+} + {}^{\cdot}O_2^{-} \rightarrow Fe^{2+} + O_2$.

The second step is the Fenton reaction: $Fe^{2+} + H_2O_2 \rightarrow Fe^{3+} + OH^{-} + {}^{\cdot}OH$.

Net reaction: ${}^{\cdot}O_2^{-} + H_2O_2 \rightarrow {}^{\cdot}OH + OH^{-} + O_2$.

And OS created by excess hydroxyl radicals (${}^{\cdot}OH$), superoxide ($O_2^{\cdot -}$), reactive non-radical compounds including singlet oxygen (${}^1O_2$), hydrogen peroxide (H_2O_2), lipid hydroperoxides, hypochlorous acid (HOCl), chloramines (RNHCl), and ozone (O_3) [11, 12] potentiates malarial infection patency and snowballing risk for fulminant disease. In the non-immune individuals, cell-mediated immune response is the initial defense mechanism which generates OS as well and subsequently, aberrant immune system response with disease traction increases.

Reactive nitrogen radical compounds such as nitric oxide (${}^{\cdot}NO$), nitrogen dioxide (${}^{\cdot}NO_2$), and non-radical nitrogen-based compounds which include peroxynitrite ($ONOO^{-}$) and dinitrogen trioxide (N_2O_3), make up the collective group of reactive nitrogen species (RNS). The unpaired electrons in their outer electron obit make these species very unstable and highly reactive. Reactive nitrogen species have direct linkages to ROS, especially in the formation of $ONOO^{-}$ which gives rise to nitrosative stress (NS).

The combination of OS and NS have been associated with the etiology of an extensive variety of disease processes and states to include aging, infections, ischemia-reperfusion (I/R) injury [13], acute kidney injury (AKI) and chronic kidney diseases [14], diabetic neuropathies [15], inflammatory disease [16], vascular dysfunction and hypertension [17], atherosclerosis, neurological diseases [18] including Alzheimer's disease [19, 20]. Most of these conditions and diseases are displayed as syndromes and facets of malaria disease.

Management of malaria, will of necessity therefore, require the inclusion of anti-disease remedies that will concurrently suppress or eradicate the pathophysiology associated with malarial. There have been strides to invent remedial treatment for malaria by improving the potency of current antimalarials. However, this avenue does not correspond to requirement of ameliorating the disease aspect of malaria. Phytochemicals, some in basic research stage of investigation or clinical stages, show promising outcomes that are worth promulgating, formulating and pre-empting strides towards attempts to eradicate both the parasite and the sequalae of malaria.

1.1 Malaria causes

There are five main Phylum Apicomplexa (Sporozoa) *Plasmodium* strains inflicting human malarial infection with changing disease outcomes, mainly *P. falciparum*, *P. vivax*, *P. malariae*, *P. ovale* and a zoonotic parasite *P. knowlesi*. Accordingly, parasite species, sub-species, host genetics and host demographics at point of infection, determine malaria disease presentations of varying intensities [21]. A disease process and time-lines with differing syndromic mediators is generated [22, 23]. The *P. falciparum* infection has the highest fatalities with strains having developed multidrug resistance. Artemisinin derivatives are the latest additions to the rug-casualties list. *P. vivax* and *P. ovale* present chronic disease with quiescent liver stage parasite hypnozoites driving disease relapses onwards of 7 years duration from initial infection reported [24]. However, there is divergent of opinion straying from this recrudescence dogma [25].

1.2 Phenotypic presentations of malaria

Malaria disease displays manifestations in adults from non-endemic areas as a different disease phenotype when compared to pregnant women and to children under the age of 5-years. Accordingly, the pathophysiology of malaria, or malaria disease [26] displays immunological idiosyncrasies, inflammatory aberrations, haemolysis which may lead to severe malaria anemia (SMA) [27], acute kidney injury (AKI) [28], and malaria cachexia leading to cardiac failure [29], hypoglycaemia [30, 31], acute respiratory distress syndrome (ARDS) [32], acute lung injury (ALI) [33], cerebral malaria [34], hyperlactaemia with non-respiratory acidosis. Of these pathophysiology, children invariably develop SMA [35], hypoglycaemia [36], hyperlactaemia with non-respiratory acidosis and cerebral malaria while adults presents with severe malaria, AKI [37] and non-respiratory acidosis [38]. Pregnant women present with placental malaria with SMA also a common feature [39]. The bottom line to all these manifestations is the OS mediation to the disease process driven by various species emanating from the parasite-human host interactions. The perceived relationship between the antioxidant capacities displayed by phytochemicals and phytotherapeutics and the oxidant-driven malaria disease motivates this chapter.

2. Malarial systemic disease and phytochemicals administration

The terms phytotherapeutics, phytotherapeutics are commonly used in the branch of science involved in the use of plant natural products and their derivatives and their use as disease management alternatives and ameliorates. The discovery that phytochemicals like the artemisinin, asiatic acid (AA), oleanolic acid and masilinic acid (MA) have both anti-inflammatory (and other physiological influences) activity and antimalarial activities have led to the exploration of their anti-disease action in malaria.

3. Oxidative stress and artemisinin malarial treatment

Artemisinin is a tetracyclic 1,2,4-trioxane containing an endoperoxide bridge (C—O—O—C), the key pharmacophore of the antimalarial [40] (**Figure 1**). Increasing solubility and pharmacological of the drug has been achieved when semi-synthetic compounds were synthesized through modification of C10 in the

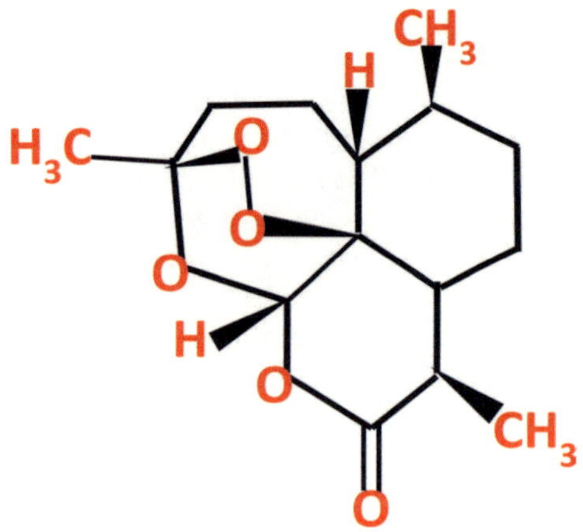

Figure 1.
Artemisinin, structure of the endoperoxides [42].

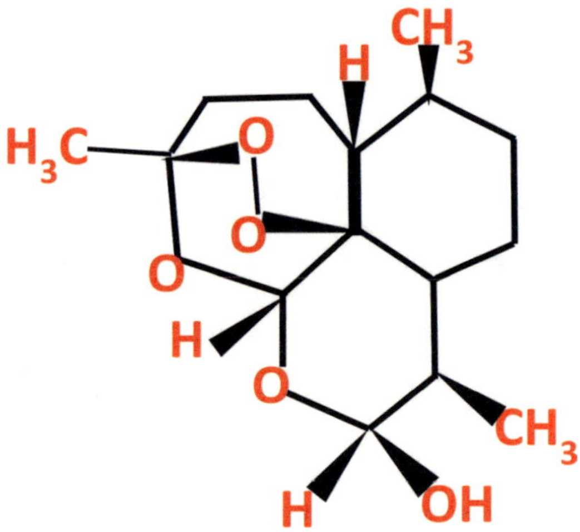

Figure 2.
Dihydroartemisinin, structure of the endoperoxides [42].

original backbone to generate hemi-acetal or ester derivative such as dihydroartemisinin (**Figure 2**), artemether (**Figure 3**) and artesunate (**Figure 4**) [41].

The debate remains unresolved on the mode(s) of activation and consequent biological target(s) of endoperoxides [43]. Activation of the endoperoxide bridge is believed to be the source of artemisinin antimalarial activity. Cleavage of the bridge, which is located at the core of the structure, generates short-lived cytotoxic oxyradicals in the presence of haem iron or free iron Fe^{2+} [44, 45]. However, two different mechanisms of action premised on the endoperoxide bioactivation, have been proposed.

Rearrangement of the oxygen-centred radicals, to produce more stable carbon-centred radicals, have been hypothesized by the Poster Laboratory using 18O-labeled trioxane analogues [46, 47]. The 'reductive scission' model, has ferrous iron binding to either O1 or O2 cleaving the endoperoxide bond and generating oxyradical intermediates which subsequently rearrange to primary or secondary carbon-centred radicals via either b-scission or a [1,5]-H shift. This hypothesis has been supported through evidence of the formation of these carbon-centred radical intermediates using electron paramagnetic resonance spin-trapping techniques [48, 49].

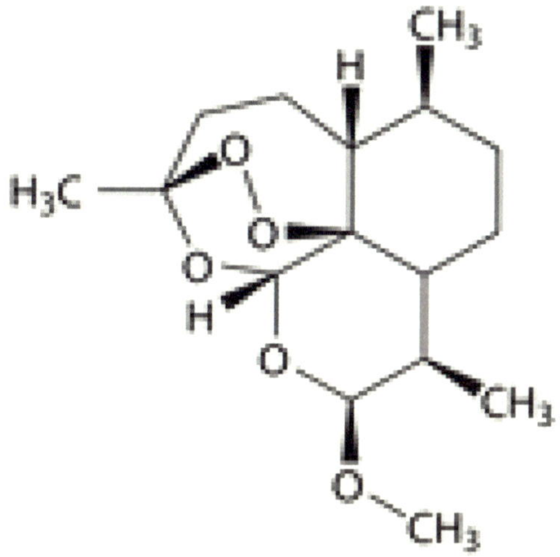

Figure 3.
Artemether, structure of the endoperoxides [42].

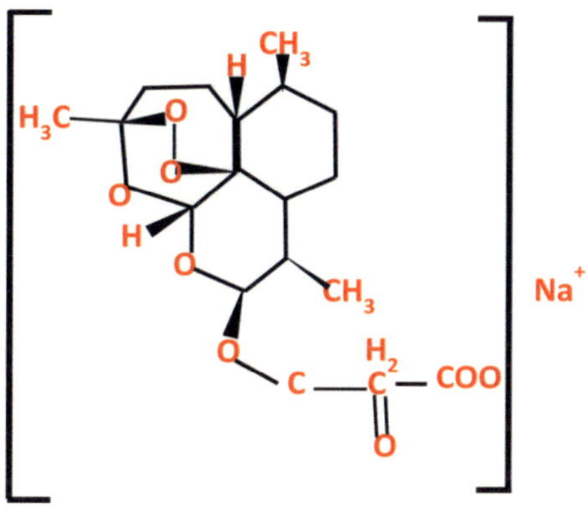

Figure 4.
Artesunate, structure of the endoperoxides [42].

Capabilities of the C-centred radicals to drive haem and or proteins alkylation have been proposed. However, the only evidence, so far provided, has been for haem alkylation [50] and a few reported model studies on protein alkylation with ferrous salts reactions in the presence of cysteine (iron-sulfur chelates) [51].

The concept of free radical generation and protein alkylation points towards creation of OS as the parasite killing apparatus of the artemisinin derivatives but also indicates the deleterious effect of the drugs on the human host and possibility of initiating or exacerbating malarial disease in the course antiparasitic activity. However, paradoxically artemisinin has been reported to be pluripotent with anti-inflammatory activity [52] although post treatment artemisinin haemolysis has also been observed in people that would have been cleared of malaria. The latter adverse reaction has been seen several weeks after successful treatment with artemisinin drugs.

3.1 Artemisinin and anti-oxidative stress disease inductions

Artemisinin and its derivatives require conversion to the biologically active dihydroartemisinin (DHA **Figure 2**) to exert their activity. Besides the excellent antimalarial effects, there is clinical and experimental evidence that suggests potent immune-suppressive against autoimmune and allergic disease of artemisinin and its derivatives [52]. Derivatives of artemisinin possessing lower range toxicity, higher bioavailability, and compelling immunosuppressive activity have been studied and some commercialized. These are 3-(12-β-artemisininoxy) phenoxyl succinic acid (SM735) [53], 1-(12-β-dihydroartemisinoxy)-2-hydroxy-3-tert-butylaminopropane maleate (SM905) [54, 55], ethyl 2-[4-(12-β-artemisininoxy)] phenoxylpropionate (SM933) [56], and 2′-aminoarteether (β)maleate (SM934) [57, 58].

To date, it is generally accepted that artemisinin wields antimalarial properties through (i) haeme or free iron breaking the peroxide bridge resulting in the degradation of artemisinin molecular structure to form the nucleophilic radical metabolite with the centre at C4. (ii) subsequently, the free radical, acting as an alkylating agent, will attack macromolecular bearing electrophilic groups or centres, which ultimately leads to parasitic demise [50, 59]. In fact, the pRBC's have increased concentrations of OS due to the parasitic infection by *Plasmodium*. In the intervening time, OS driven free radicals and lipid peroxidation concentrations dramatically increase intracellularly. Apparently, pRBC's are rendered more susceptible to artemisinin than npRBC's. In vivo artemisinin is effective in killing pRBC's at nM concentrations which differs sharply when contrasted to marginal effects of artemisinin on resting RBC's even at high mM concentrations [60, 61].

3.2 Anti-inflammation and immunoregulatory effect of artemisinin

There are three fundamental steps by which T cells perform pivotal role in acquired immune reaction [62, 63]: (i) G0 to G1 transition of T cells is driven by TCR cross-linking which leads to the secretion of T cell growth factor IL-2 and expression of high-affinity receptor IL-2Rα chain (CD25); (ii) through autocrine and or paracrine proliferative loop, IL-2 influences clone expansion and maintains activated T cells survival; (iii) after efficacious clearance of the pathogen, the inducement for cytokines production is lost and activated T cells will undergo apoptosis.

Nevertheless, in autoimmune diseases, due to the tenacity of autoantigen, autoreactive T cells will be activated and with better survival [52]. Autoreactive T cell proliferation is involved in the pathogenesis of various immune-related diseases, such as rheumatoid arthritis (RA) and multiple sclerosis (MS) [20, 21] as well as malaria.

Artemether is a powerful antimalarial drug [64] found to significantly suppress the proliferation and synthesis of IL-2 and interferon-γ (IFN-γ) by T cells through the TCR engagement influence [65]. The TCR engagement-triggered MAPKs signaling pathway as well as phosphorylation of ERK1/2, Jnk, and P38 were significantly inhibited by artemether. Discovery was made that artemether greatly affects T cells function as compared to that of the antigen presenting cells (APCs) to exert the immunosuppressive effects [65].

A series of artemisinin derivatives, with higher water solubility and lower toxicity, have been created by inserting, to the parent artemisinin structure, new functional groups like ethylene glycol [66, 67]. These have immunosuppressive targeted at T cell activation suppression, combat inflammation through substantial inhibition of the proliferation and production of IFN-γ, IL-12 and IL-6. While there is no direct influence of artemether and its derivatives on IL-2 and CD25 upregulation of T cells, there is remarkable suppression of IL-2-mediated proliferation and survival of activated T cells alluding to blocking of IL-2 induced phosphorylation of Akt [68]. Additionally, artemether derivative SM934-driven preferential early apoptosis activated of T cells, with no effect on resting T cells, has been observed through staining of CD69 and annexin V.

Furthermore, studies suggesting that artemisinin derivatives bind to calmodulin to inhibit phosphodiesterase activity, which causes the increase of intracellular cAMP concentration, and therefore to exert the immunosuppressive activity have been reported [69, 70].

Additionally, oral treatment of SM905 has been shown to skew the T cell subset from pathogenic Th17 to protective Th2 subset in an arthritic model with increased IL-4 production and suppression of the RORγt mRNA expression together with IL-17 production [71]. The artemisinin derivatives' effects hinge on the anti-inflammatory properties which play an antimalarial role. To back this assertion up, artesunate has minor effects on inflammatory responses downstream of antibody production demonstrating that highly proliferative germinal centre B cells are the most sensitive cellular targets to the treatment. Significantly, *in vitro* artesunate inhibits IL-1β, IL-6, and IL-8 production by way of stimulation by TNF-α as well as the expression of vascular endothelial growth factor and hypoxia-inducible factor-1α [72]. Moreover, artesunate inhibits Akt phosphorylation and IκB degradation by blocking PI3K/Akt signaling pathway downstream of TNF-α [73] making it an efficient adjunct to malarial inflammatory response characterized by increased and decreased Th1 and Th2 type cytokines, respectively.

The intriguing anti-inflammatory properties of the artemisinin (SM933) are observed through the regulatory mechanism involving the NFκB and Rig-G/JAB1 pathways which regulation alters cell cycle activity of activated T cells selectively. In contrast to SM933, SM934 and DHA treatment is majorly through the regulation of the balance between effector T cells and regulatory T cells. Administering of DHA significantly decreases effectors CD4 T cells and increases in Treg cells in a reciprocal regulatory process through modulation of the mTOR pathway which characterizes its regulatory mechanism [56, 74].

3.3 Artemisinin structure: activity relationship in oxidative stress

Macromolecules bearing electrophilic groups or centres are prone to alkylating nucleophilic radicals, metabolites of artemisinin, which eventually leads to cell damages [61]. Furthermore, artemisinin inhibits endoplasmic reticulum Ca^{2+} ATPase (SERCA) with consequent cytoplasmic calcium accumulation and secondary activation of cellular calcium influx. In this way artemisinin induces *P. falciparum* cellular apoptosis [75]. The same effect has been shown by thapsigargin (TG), a specific SERCA inhibitor with structural similarity to artemisinin, which induces cellular calcium accumulation leading to apoptosis. While artemisinin and TG have the same binding sites on SERCA, there are structural biology differences in the binding pocket for different mammalian and *Plasmodium* species resultantly conferring differential susceptibility to the drug. A single amino acid (Leu263) in the transmembrane segment 3 of SERCA in *P. vivax* SERCA (PvCERCA) has a 3-fold sensitivity to artemisinin while introduction of the same residue in *P. berghei* SERCA (PbSERCA) decreases sensitivity 3-fold [75, 76].

Interestingly, while the peroxide bridge plays a necessary role in the artemisinin biological activity, artemisinin-SERCA binding does not involve this moiety [77] but play a catalytic role in the inhibition [52]. Naturally, stereochemistry and transitional state theory have it that the intact peroxide bridge makes the spatial configuration of artemisinin to be relatively rigid and making the sesquiterpene lactone unable to flexibly rotate and fold. This results in lower affinity for SERCA. Reduction and breaking of the peroxide bridge by divalent iron ion, however, releases the sesquiterpene lactone increasing its flexibility and binding affinity to SERCA enhancing inhibitory effect of artemisinin on the enzyme. Moreover, the concentration of Fe^{2+} in pRBC's and activated lymphocytes is significantly increased compared to resting state cells increasing the opportunity for peroxide bridge to be broken. In this manner, the pRBC's and activated leukocytes, rather than npRBC's and resting cells, become more vulnerable to artemisinin activity. Nevertheless, the mammalian SERCA is not susceptible to artemisinin inhibition [75]. Therefore, the biochemical mechanism and artemisinin molecular target to exert immunosuppression in malaria and other disease driven by OS requires further perusal and investigations.

4. Asiatic acid (AA) administration and oxidative stress-driven malarial disease

Asiatic acid (AA), in **Figure 2**, is a naturally occurring pentacyclic triterpenoid originating from the herb *Centella asiatica*. Triterpenoid saponins are the primary constituents of *C. asiatica* responsible for extensive therapeutic actions. The molecular mechanisms underlying the various biological activities of AA have been described for malarial diseases as it is driven by OS. The pharmacological properties of AA and its derivatives inhibit multiple pathways of intracellular signaling molecules and transcription factors that are involved in the various stages of acute and chronic diseases [78]. The anti-inflammatory [79], anti-hyperlipidemia, malarial hypoglycaemia ameliorative effective [30], neuroprotective, reno-protective effects [80] and other activities of AA have an intricate and elaborate pattern, amongst the triterpenes, that is envisaged on the pleiotropic characteristics bed rocked on its anti-oxidative pro-oxidative properties and redox reactivity [81, 82].

4.1 Severe malaria anemia (SMA) and anti-disease effects of asiatic acid activity

One of the major causes of morbidity and mortality in malaria is SMA driven by a multifaceted etiology. Noteworthy mechanisms contributing to SMA include (i) increased destruction of pRBC's and npRBC's (immune system mediated haemolysis, phagocytosis, splenic sequestration); (ii) decreased RBC's synthesis from immune system and parasite effects [83, 84]. The number of RBC's turnover is a balanced process under normal physiology and a decrease in concentration (anemia) is predicted by an efflux of reticulocytes from hematopoietic tissues. When anemia develops from increased RBC's destruction, such as haemolysis or hemorrhage, erythropoietin (EPO) production in kidneys is normally up-regulated with a concomitant increase in reticulocytosis to alleviate rheological disturbances. Together with EPO, growth factors and cytokines, to include granulocyte colony-stimulating factor (G-SF), stem cell factor (SF), insulin-like growth fator-1 (IGF-1), take active involvement in erythropoiesis [85, 86].

Therefore, production of EPO in the peritubular fibroblasts of the renal cortex, requires that the kidneys physiology be normal [87, 88] and is determined by the amount of oxygen present which depends on the concentration of RBC's. Tissue oxygen tension and hypoxia regulates EPO production in a feed-back loop with hematocrit, centred on an inverse logarithmic relationship [89]. Increased hypoxia resulting from SMA causes increased OS. Therefore, antioxidant capacity of AA is able to correct hematocrit and ameliorating SMA [26]. However, the principle by which this effect of AA on OS in SMA is premised on its effect in reducing kidney lipid peroxidation and increasing antioxidant defenses in malaria.

This has a positive effect on oxygen tension and EPO production [90]. Overall, OS driven by SMA revolves around hypoxia which emanates from reduced oxygen delivery due to reduced RBC's mass exacerbated by dysfunctional EPO synthesis.

Correction of both OS and SMA, as does AA, is pivotal to malarial disease amelioration and resolution through modulation of the immune system responses.

4.2 Immune system as mediator of SMA generation

While the immune system plays a fundamental part in erythropoiesis, in SMA, the immune response is central to its pathogenesis with pRBC's, hemozoin, and glycosylphosphatidylinositol (GPI) which activates monocyte and lymphocyte singly or jointly followed by increased inflammatory mediator synthesis. Pro-inflammatory mediators TNF-α, TNF-γ, IL-1 and IL-23 tend to be up-regulated while anti-inflammatory cytokines IL-4 and IL-10 exhibit low concentrations in SMA [91, 92]. The over expression of Th1 cytokines in malaria and SMA invariably affects erythropoiesis negatively and enhance OS. There is a close association between macrophage inhibiting factor (MIF) and SMA with bone marrow (BM) activity suppression influenced by NO as a powerful erythropoiesis inhibitor [93, 94]. Haemolysis and associated *Plasmodium* products like hemozoin intrinsically motivates SMA, erythropoiesis dysfunction, vasoconstriction which perturbs inducible nitric oxide synthase (iNOS) and increased EPO compensatory increases. However, increased EPO concentrations convoyed by insufficient erythroid progenitors response results in low reticulocytotic presentations [92, 95]. Ultimately, ineffective erythropoiesis, erythrophagocytosis and iron delocalisation may have a bearing on SMA [96]. Taken together, inflammatory responses and OS, which are corrected by AA administration, have a strong bearing in SMA outcomes.

Transdermal delivery of AA, as a once off application of a pectin hydrogel patch, influences hematocrit (Hct), a surrogate marker for SMA, suggests the phytochemical has influence on some yet unidentified mechanism of red blood cell (RBC) molecular level metabolism [79]. By influencing the causes of low Hct and SMA, which could be increased parasitaemia induced-haemolysis or inflammation induced-erythropoiesis-suppression, AA is able to address reduced RBC's concentration of malaria. Inflammation drives OS (and vice versa) and its attending outcomes through well-established mechanisms involving cytokines and other soluble effector molecules in a vicious cycle.

The TNF-α and other cytokines are well established inflammatory mediators. Reports of AA inhibition of TNF-α in acute pancreatitis in corneal lipoploysaccharide induced inflammation have been made. The phytochemical's antinociceptive activities and anti-inflammation in mice has been linked to its ability to inhibit cytokine activity [97–99]. Ultrasensitive fourth generation CRP concentrations have been shown to be significantly lower in *P. berghei* (murine malaria)-infected rats administered with both oral and transdermal amidated hydrogel matrix pectin patch as compared to untreated animals. This indicates an anti-inflammatory effect of the phytochemical [79] which is an essential anti-disease effect in malaria through inhibition of inflammatory markers like TNF-α.

Nonetheless, it has been shown that TNF-α causes hypoferraemia and reduces intestinal absorption of iron [100, 101]. A strong influence of SMA generation has been shown by increased concentrations of the cytokine in malaria [102] with a distinct mechanism for inadequate erythropoiesis linked to the cytokine [103]. Inflammation is a crucial driver of malaria where TNF-α is a key component, and SMA is a common complication [104] through erythropoiesis perturbations [105]. Therefore, it stands to reason that AA's influence on both inflammation and SMA could be through inhibition of TNF-α as an association between suppression of the cytokine by the phytochemical has been observed.

As a result, the relationship between AA and TNF-α in malaria present key proponents to malaria disease management. Notwithstanding, a similarly structured triterpene, oleanolic acid (OA), has been reported to attenuate pro-inflammatory cytokines (TNF-α and IL-6) release and ameliorate anemia in murine malaria [106], properties that AA has been reported to have in other inflammatory conditions [107].

Ferroportin (FPN), an abundant protein in the reticuloendothelial system which mediates iron release and intestinal iron absorption, has its cytoplasm re-localisation induced by TNF-α [108]. This effect is obtained through working in tandem with hepcidin which is abundantly expressed in malaria and other chronic diseases with concomitant EPO resistance and dyserythropoiesis [109, 110]. Thus, possible inhibition of TNF-α and the known amelioration of anemia in malaria by AA may positively influence TNF-α-induced hypoferraemia which is driven by inflammatory mediators on hepcidin [101].

4.3 Ferroportin (FPN) and SMA

Interestingly, FPN expression on RBC's (54,000 copies per cell) has been reported as a novel finding for a protein that had not been thought to be found on these cells as export of Fe^{2+} had been thought to occur only after haemolysis of pRBC's [111]. By the exportation of iron generated by hemoglobin autoxidation, FPN protects against iron accumulation, as well as malaria infection and haemolysis creating an antioxidation status in the cell. In situations where there is increased inflammation, increases hepcidin synthesis which dysregulates FPN metabolism and increases Fe^{2+} accumulation within both the pRBC's and npRBC's promotes iron deficiency and haemolysis from OS [112]. The ability of AA to ameliorate malaria-associated inflammation and OS is critical in to the phytochemical's salvaging of Hct and SMA through preservation and or upregulation of FPN activity in both pRBC's and npRBC's. By reducing cellular Fe^{2+} in pRBC's parasites proliferation intracellularly is inhibited and protection against the disease conferred. Iron supplementation in malaria down-regulates FPN influencing growth of the parasite worsening malaria [113, 114]. Upregulation of FPN by AA is a possible mechanism by which the phytotherapeutic effects antiparasitic activity and anti-disease in murine malaria.

4.4 The inflammasome in chronic disease and asiatic acid administration

The inflammasome, a key component in the development of chronic disease anemia is characterized by anemia and decrease in RBC's volume corresponding with the patent period of murine malaria infection. During the patent period, rapid parasite multiplication is experienced culminating in peak parasitaemia and death. However, timely intervention with AA administration as a chemoprophylactic has salvages Sprague-Dawley (SD) rats from the brink of death to full recovery with 0% parasitaemia at Day 12–15 post infection [26].

Peak parasitaemia effects on infection outcomes are compounded by suboptimal EPO directed responses such as reduced cellular proliferation (with adequate EPO production) to SMA. The inflammasome seem to be the major underlying factor driving tissue insensitivity to EPO which leads to SMA even in acute cases. Administration of AA to reverses this process by restoring normal hemoglobin (Hb) concentrations and Hct.

4.5 Inflammasome drives SMA through hepcidin-ferroportin influence

Iron metabolism is influenced by inflammation of chronic disease through hepcidin, the inhibitor of the only known iron exporter. Inflammation drives the synthesis of hepcidin in the liver with cytokines TNF-α, IL-1 and IL-6 playing a major role. Interestingly, the hepcidin phenomenon, by driving reduction in iron concentrations, is calculated to protect against severe *P. falciparum* malaria and death in young children [113]. Iron deficiency has also been shown to have a 5.5-fold protection against placental malaria fatalities [115]. Modulation of Fe^{2+} concentration resulting in iron deficiency uses hepcidin synthesis in chronic inflammation of malaria. This, therefore, means that inhibition of inflammation mediators will also influence hepcidin synthesis and thus remove the metabolic barricade on iron export by FPN.

The pleiotropic nature of AA comes to the fore in its ability to attenuate inflammatory cytokines (TNF-α. IL-1, IL-6) and combat malarial parasitaemia as well as influence iron metabolism through hepcidin. A direct causal relationship between hepcidin is and AA is yet to be established. However, it stands to reason that if AA is able to attenuate the drivers of hepcidin synthesis, it is also able to influence the hormone's metabolism. Subsequently AA may be able to influence iron metabolism through the same process of FPN-hepcidin interaction and reduction of iron export from enterocytes, macrophages, hepatocytes and RBC's. Preservation and recovery of SMA evidenced by normalization of Hct and other RBC indices (reported elsewhere) in malaria and parasitaemia reduction by AA indicates the possibility of its influence on FPN effects on iron export lost in pRBC's and was recovered for normal intracellular iron to take place.

There is an abundance of FPN on RBCs with effects on RBC iron status, and when down-regulated by hepcidin [111, 112] or other inhibitor could therefore influence the growth of malaria parasites [116, 117]. However, FPN down-regulation in malaria mediates parasitaemia proliferation, increase intracellular OS from accumulation of haeme Fe^{2+} [111]. The mutation of FPN Q24H (glutamine to histidine switch at position 248) is prevalent in sub-Saharan Africa populations with a prevalence of between 2.2–20% [118, 119] renders FPN resistant to hepcidin-induced degradation [120]. Due to the nonregulated form of the FPN, carriers tend to have lower hemoglobin concentrations than normal controls which is consistent with findings that high FPN levels in erythroblasts tend to export more iron, diminish hemoglobin synthesis [121, 122] although it may have protective effect against OS as a health benefit to those of African descent. Phytochemical administration in malaria and their effects on hepcidin-ferroportin relationship may have the same effect.

4.6 Mechanisms of oxidative stress, haemolysis and SMA in malaria

The underlying cause of malarial anemia does not get fully explained by dyserythropoiesis as it may have a rapid onset and life-threatening outcomes. A plausible explanation of reduced RBC mass includes the haemolysis associated with both pRBC's and npRBC's that occurs in malaria through changes that take place in the cell membranes.

While in the circulation, RBC's are in constant exposure to endogenous and exogenous reactive OS (ROS) with a high potential for cell damage and functional impairment through OS. However, ROS effects are minimized by the extensive antioxidant system involving non-enzymatic antioxidants of low molecular weight (glutathione and ascorbic acids as examples) and enzymatic antioxidants like superoxide dismutase, catalase, [123] glutathione reductase [124], and peroxiredoxin-2 [125, 126]. These antioxidants preserve the life span of RBC's through preserving cell membrane integrity [127]. The antioxidant ability to neutralize endogenous ROS is diminished when the blood flows through the microcirculation when hemoglobin (Hb) becomes partially oxygenated [128], more so in malaria-infection cells. Also, partial oxygenation consequence in conformational changes of Hb and a dramatic increase in autoxidation of Hb building up with attending OS [129, 130]. Un-neutralized ROS in the RBC causes membrane damage that impairs their flow through the microcirculation and oxygen delivery to the tissues inducing hypoxia and OS generation [131]. Also, cells that come in contact with RBC's containing increased ROS tend to receive OS with subsequent tissue damage and inflammation induction [132, 133]. Indications are that RBC's NADH oxidase generate ROS from their membrane locations [134] away from the reach of cytoplasmic antioxidant enzymes.

One other none Hb autoxidation related OS leading to RBC deformity is associated with caspase 3. In the RBC, caspase 3 is activated by oxidative reactions with resultant degradation of band 3 [135, 136] which induce the exposure of phosphatidylserine, usually located in the inner leaflet of RBC membrane, to the outer surface [137]. The resultant histrionic reorganization of the membrane is concomitant with decrease in the discoid cell deformability [138] and ultimate haemolysis and RBC's mass reduction.

4.6.1 Oxidative stress, ATPases interaction and SMA

Ionic movement and homeostasis play a critical role in the development of OS and ensuing sequalae driving SMA. Inhibition of Ca^{2+}ATPase by OS [139, 140] enhances intracellular calcium concentration and activity with resultant RBC deformability decreases. Deregulated intracellular calcium concentration tend to activate the Gardos channel that results in potassium leakage from the RBC with subsequent cation homeostasis destabilization [128, 141] and shrinkage of cell with impaired deformability [128].

In malaria the total antioxidant capacity is compromised in the later stages of erythrocytic parasite development with membrane damage and breeches occurring through increased OS in both in npRBC's and pRBC's leading to SMA [142] as the RBC seem to be the readily available ROS sink in the disease [2]. This contributes to premature RBC's senescence and poor deformability resulting in the cells' splenic entrapment in the complex macrophage-abundant red pulp fenestrations [142, 143]. Oxidative stress is also associated with increased cell volume and density [144]. The growing parasite also increases OS and cell density that causes RBC microvesiculation as deformability and flexibility decreases exponentially. Any alterations that affects RBC volume and excess surface area tend to affect deformability of the cell [128] and this is a common occurrence in malaria leading to haemolysis, RBC concentration and SMA.

By interfering with parasite proliferation in murine malaria, AA directly contributes to normalizing cell volume and surface areas which aspects preserves cellular morphology in malaria [79, 145].

The induction of inducible nitric oxide synthase (iNOS), which increases NO synthesis, is closely linked to the inflammatory response in malaria with vascular permeability, pulmonary oedema and SMA as outcomes [146]. Increasing NO synthesis causes inhibition of the Na^+/K^+ ATPase with subsequent disturbance of water homeostasis in both the npRBC's, pRBC's and other tissues [147, 148]. When ATPase pump fails there is an accumulation of Na^+ in the intracellular compartment of both npRBC's and pRBC's with ensuing increased cell volume and surface area, membrane rigidity and reduced deformability and infiltrability in the spleen. Concomitant to decreased RBC's filterability is their removal by the spleen leading to SMA [27, 149]. ROS and $ONOO^-$ from inflammatory processes of malaria may have the same effect through oxidation of cell membranes and inhibition of the Na^+/K^+ ATPase pump with consequential SMA [150, 151]. Notwithstanding ATPase inhibition, universal ATP depletion in malaria also uncouples the enzymes followed by RBC's membrane deformities, haemolysis and acute SMA [96, 152].

The fundamental basis of SMA driven by npRBC's and pRBC's spleen sequestration is underpinned by a synergistic effect of inflammation, OS (ROS and NS) and ATP depletion, falls under the ambit of disease processes resolved by the pleiotropic AA through its anti-inflammatory, antioxidant and neuroprotective roles [97, 107, 153]. There is an intriguing coordination of immune and erythropoietic responses in malaria related OS played by the AA administration which speculates extra dimensions in controlling parasitaemia and alleviation of SMA.

4.7 Malarial hypoglycaemia expression and the oxidative stress phenotype

Childhood *P. falciparum* malaria syndrome is preceded by a strong expression of hypoglycaemia. The etiology of low glucose concentrations in malaria have been accredited to antimalarial drugs like quinine and chloroquine which exhibit insulinomimetic action although patients without either intervention or disease have shown incapacitating hypoglycaemia [154]. Low blood sugar in malaria has also been attributed to increased consumption by growing parasites, but hypoglycaemia has been reported in low parasite loads in humans and it has also been shown that parasite only consume about 10% of the total plasma glucose even in severe malaria [155, 156].

A good and well characterized correlation exists in malaria between hyperlactaemia, hypoglycaemia and parasitaemia [157]. The possibility of microvasculature obstruction contributing to tissue hypoxia with attendant inefficient glucose utilization is plausible. Nevertheless, annotations that normal overall blood flow in the brain during periods of coma in malaria have been indicated [158]. Low blood flow rates in areas adjacent to high blood flow areas may elucidate the anomaly, however, hyperlactaemia requires a different explanation than the microcirculation obstruction alone and most likely a synergy with cytokine-induced oxygen underutilization could be involved [159, 160]. Elevated TNF-α has been associated with hypoglycaemia, hyperlactaemia and non-respiratory acidosis (nRA) in a number of diseases not related to malaria microvasculature obstruction as well [161]. Deliberate intervention with TNF-α in animals models tend to induce the same parameters [162, 163].

A causal relationship of hypoglycaemia and TNF-α may be intimated in malaria [164]. *Borrelia recurrentis* infection tends to elevate TNF-α in association with inflammation and the triumvirate of hypoglycaemia, non-respiratory acidosis and hyperlactaemia although there will not be parasites to excrete lactate or cause microvasculature occlusion [165].

Overall, TNF-α seem to be the main orchestrator of inflammation and that the anti-inflammatory effects of AA through inhibition of inflammatory mediators influence hypoglycaemia amelioration in malaria [30]. Indeed, the biologically active pentacyclictriterpenoid compounds oleanolic acid (OA) and maslinic acid (MA) have been shown to clear parasitic infection and ameliorate hypoglycaemia associated with malaria [106, 166] (**Figure 5**).

Asiatic acid and MA influence on glucose homeostasis in murine malaria involves the attenuation of glycolytic hormone activity by, in part, inhibiting glycogen phosphorylase (GP). Asiatic acid binds at the allosteric activator site naturally occupied the physiological activator AMP [30, 167]. This way glycolytic oxidation of glucose is reduced through reduced substrate while glycogen synthesis is upregulated. Mitochondrial associated OS may be reduced by inhibiting GP, as happens with glycogen synthase kinase 3β inhibition in chronic myocardial ischaemia or hypoxia [168], under hypoglycaemic conditions of malaria that would have rather increase glucose mobilization being the norm. Actually, glycogen stores tend to be high in animals that are administered with AA as compared to non-treated controls, in experiments mentioned above showing glycogen preservation [30]. Inactivation of GP not only reduce glycogenolysis but also stimulates glycogen synthesis [167] preserving normoglycaemia in malaria and normoinsulinism. **Figure 6** indicates the allosteric binding site for the inhibitor AA on the dimeric GP.

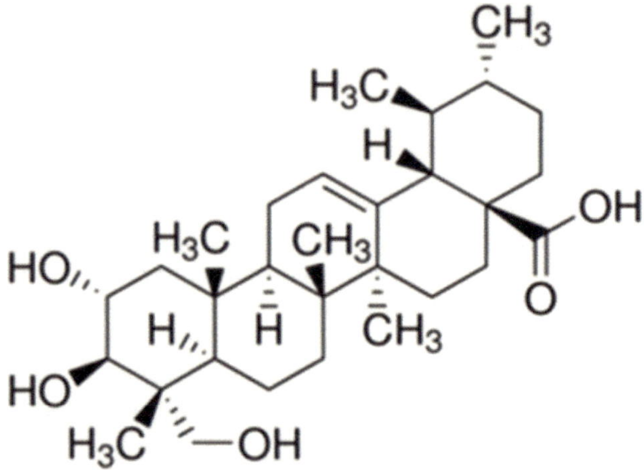

Figure 5.
Asiatic acid.

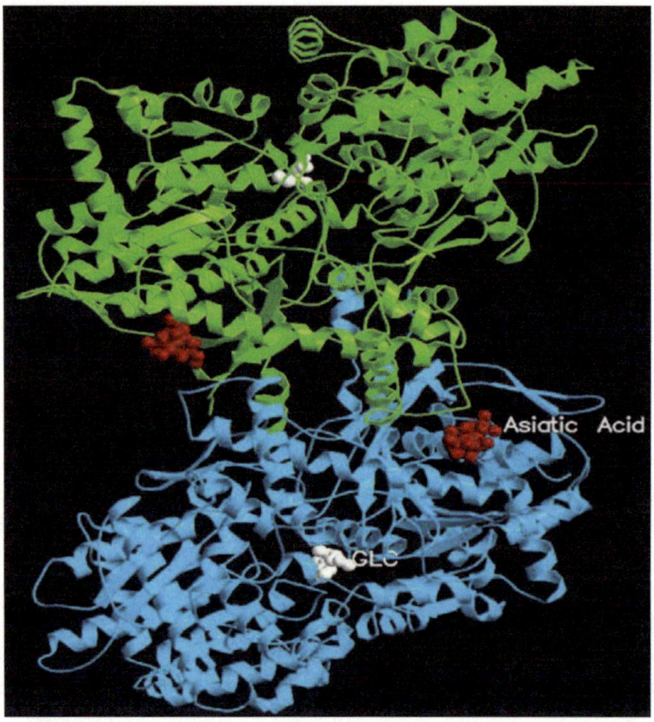

Figure 6.
Schematic diagram of the glycogen phosphorylase dimeric molecule, for residues 10–837, viewed down the molecular dyad. The catalytic (marked by GLUCOSE in white) and the allosteric (binds AMP and the inhibitors AA shown in red) binding sites positions are indicated. The allosteric site is situated at the subunit-subunit interface some 30 Å from the catalytic site [167].

The *Plasmodium* parasite, immunological and inflammatory responses, as well as chemotherapeutics currently used cause hypoglycaemia in malaria. The anti-hyperglycaemic, antioxidant, pro-oxidant properties useful in glucose homeostasis, observed when AA is administered in malaria, is hinged possibly on its influence on controlling hormonal as well as enzymatic aberrations seen in malaria and its treatment as explained above, where chloroquine and quinine treatment of malaria has been implicated with hyperinsulinism driving hypoglycaemia [169, 170].

A pre-clinical experiment showed that insulin resistance, which invariably causes hyperinsulinism [171], was ameliorated after administration of AA in malaria [30]. Oral administration of AA at 10 mg kg maintained normoinsulinism with reciprocal activity of glucagon in murine malaria in this study. Moreover, AA attenuated key glycolytic enzymes in streptozotocin-induced diabetes mellitus [172] an aspect that was seen in murine malaria with an overall effect on glucose tolerance response. Also, administration of AA terminated the satiation effects of high glucagon concentrations [173]. Also, positively modulated by AA administration, was the alleviation of the otherwise negative effects of malaria on food intake and weight gain.

Malaria induced-hypoxia producing hyperlactataemia was also ablated in animals that were administered with AA giving an overall high-grade wellbeing as opposed to severe malaria infection [174].

5. Malarial acute kidney injury (AKI) and oxidative stress

Kidney injury, acute or chronic, is one of the common differential diagnosis of malaria manifesting as syndrome. The diverse presentations and aetiological mechanisms of AKI orbit around the properties of pRBC's on microcirculation, hypovolaemia, metabolic derangements or host immunologic responses to infection [175–177]. These major pathogenic features are originated by the *Plasmodium* infection but may not be limited by the annihilation of the infection. Malaria associated AKI may develop after parasite abolition [178] necessitating interventions that also eradicate disease effects after parasitaemia clearance. Oxidative stress plays a critical role in AKI etiology driven by either the parasite or the immunological response to malaria infection which require neutralization in malaria. The source of kidney impairment in malaria is through direct tissue injury or inhibition of key components of kidney function. Inflammation as an immunological response initiator or vice versa has a close link to AKI development through OS initiators free haem Fe^{2+} and hemozoin which generate OS. Disruption of Na^{+} transporters by OS in the kidney [179] results in sodium wasting syndrome (hypernaturia), hypovolaemia with severe dehydration and non-respiratory acidosis leading to hyponatraemia and reduced glomerular filtration in malaria infection [180, 181] and malaria treatment with chloroquine complicates the disease [182, 183]. Therefore, renoprotective agents in the management of malaria AKI are imperative.

By combining the amphiphilic AA and amidated pectin hydrogel matrix in a transdermal drug delivery system provides a robust framework for combating malaria with renal function and electrolyte preservations [80]. AA-hydrogel matrix administration confers "an apply and walk away" once-off treatment for malaria as compared to the convoluted regimens of current antimalarial drugs in both dose, dosage frequency and administration route, not to mention the oxidative damage they bring. The non-nephrotoxicity of AA has been demonstrated in virtual screening experiments searching for selective inhibitors of 11β-hydroxysteroid dehydrogenase 1 (11β-HSD 1) against 11β-hydroxysteroid dehydrogenase 2 (11β-HSD 2) [184].

These enzymes catalyze the interconversion of cortisone and cortisol in humans [185]. The isoform 11β-HSD 1 is located in the liver, adipose and brain where it converts the inactive cortisone to the active cortisol and 11β-HSD 2 is primarily expressed in kidney catalyzing the reverse conversion. The two enzymes provide a balance in glucocorticoid metabolism. AA was shown to selectively inhibit 11β-HSD 1 and not the other isoform. When 11β-HSD 1 is inhibited there is a resultant reduction in liver gluconeogenesis, lipophilia and there is improved insulin sensitivity [186], which may explain the positive influence of AA administration on glucose homeostasis in malaria [30]. Therefore, 11β-HSD inhibition by AA works in tandem with AA glycogen phosphorylase (GP) inhibition (see above) that preserve glycogen stores. Indeed, the kidney glycogen stores tend to be significantly higher in AA administered SD rats than untreated controls. Nevertheless, inhibition of 11β-HSD 2 leads to sodium retention, hypokalemia and hypertension [187] parameters which were not observed with AA administration as compared to controls in the transdermal drug delivery of AA studies above.

Further, selective inhibition of 11β-HSD 1 has been suggested to induce anti-inflammatory effect via the stimulation of haeme oxygenase-1 in LPS-activated mice and J774.1 in murine macrophages [188], which may explain the preservation of renal electrolyte handling that was observed when AA was administered. Electrolyte loss in malaria results from inhibition of Na^+/K^+ ATPase, ENac and other electrolyte channels by OS (ROS) in the proximal convoluted tubules which results in an increased sodium load reaching the distal convoluted tubes. Excess Na^+ is as a result lost in the urine in a what is referred to as pseudohypoaldosteronism. Therefore, a dual role of AA may be observed in malarial AKI in that the anti-inflammatory and antioxidant effect through the selective inhibition of 11β-HSD 1 with ultimate reduction in gluconeogenesis which reduce glycolysis and in lipid synthesis which reduces lipid peroxidation. Antioxidant capacity is seen through AA inhibition of glycogen phosphorylase and glycolysis modulation. Increased insulin insensitivity, that is usually seen in end-stage malaria fronted by increasing glucose concentrations and OS, is abolished by AA inhibition of 11β-HSD 1. Furthermore, glycogen synthase upregulation when glycogen phosphorylase is inhibited increases glycogen storage in the kidneys and this way restoring optimum renal function and electrolyte handling deranged by OS driven AKI. Also, inhibition of 11β-HSD1 promotes autophagy and correlates with reduced OS, inflammation [189] which are key pundits in malarial AKI eradicable by AA administration.

6. Conclusion

Oxidative stress drives malaria pathophysiology by ROS and NS insults upon pRBC's and npRBC's from parasitic infection, immunological host response. The inflammatory milieu has a cross cutting foot print in malarial syndromes intricately intertwining complex disease events, processes and systems to bring about malaria disease. Here we have shown how artemisinin, a commonly used antimalarial phytotherapeutic and asiatic acid, an experimental antimalarial phytochemical, to explain their various interactions in the combat of malarial disease.

Asiatic acid, armed with constitutive antioxidant and oxidative properties inhibit parasitic growth, host inflammasome and ameliorates systemic abnormalities in malaria. With selective enzymatic inhibition propensities, apoptotic influences and amelioration of malaria-induced systemic metabolic derangements, AA shows potential as an anti-parasitic, anti-disease, anti-inflammatory, antioxidant, immunomodulatory, renoprotective and malarial disease elixir.

Abbreviations

AA	asiatic acid
ARF	acute renal failure
SMA	severe malaria anemia
nRA	non-respiratory acidosis
NO	nitric oxide
iNOS	inducible nitric oxide synthase
$ONOO^-$	peroxynitrite
ROS	reactive oxygen species
pRBC's	parasitized red blood cells
npRBC's	non-parasitized red blood cells

Author details

Greanious Alfred Mavondo[1*], Blessing Nkazimulo Mkhwanazi[2], Joy Mavondo[3], Wisdom Peresuh[4] and Obadiah Moyo[5]

1 National University of Science and Technology, Faculty of Medicine, Pathology Department, Bulawayo, Zimbabwe

2 University of KwaZulu Natal (UKZN), Pietermaritzburg, South Africa

3 Imagegate Diagnostics (PL), Bulawayo, Zimbabwe

4 Labnet Laboratories (P/L), Bulawayo, Zimbabwe

5 Chitungwiza General Hospital, Chitungwiza, Zimbabwe

*Address all correspondence to: greanious.mavondo@nust.ac.zw

References

[1] Dondorp AM, Omodeo-Salè F, Chotivanich K, Taramelli D, White NJ. Oxidative stress and rheology in severe malaria. Redox Report. 2003;**8**:292-294

[2] Becker K, Tilley L, Vennerstrom JL, Roberts D, Rogerson S, Ginsburg H. Oxidative stress in malaria parasite-infected erythrocytes: Host-parasite interactions. International Journal for Parasitology. 2004;**34**:163-189

[3] Narsaria N, Mohanty C, Das BK, Mishra SP, Prasad R. Oxidative stress in children with severe malaria. Journal of Tropical Pediatrics. 2012;**58**:147-150

[4] Potter SM, Mitchell AJ, Cowden WB, Sanni LA, Dinauer M, Haan JB, et al. Phagocyte-derived reactive oxygen species do not influence the progression of murine blood-stage malaria infections. Infection and Immunity. 2005;**73**:4941-4947

[5] Keller CC, Kremsner PG, Hittner JB, Misukonis MA, Weinberg JB, Perkins DJ. Elevated nitric oxide production in children with malarial anemia: Hemozoin-induced nitric oxide synthase type 2 transcripts and nitric oxide in blood mononuclear cells. Infection and Immunity. 2004;**72**:4868-4873

[6] Sohail M, Kaul A, Raziuddin M, Adak T. Decreased glutathione-S-transferase activity: Diagnostic and protective role in vivax malaria. Clinical Biochemistry. 2007;**40**:377-382

[7] Guha M, Kumar S, Choubey V, Maity P. Apoptosis in liver during malaria: Role of oxidative stress and implication of mitochondrial pathway. The FASEB Journal. 2006;**20**:E439-E449

[8] Kumar S, Bandyopadhyay U. Free heme toxicity and its detoxification systems in human. Toxicology Letters. 2005;**157**:175-188

[9] Koppenol WH. The Haber-Weiss cycle—70 years later. Redox Report. 2001;**6**(4):229-234. DOI: 10.1179/135100001101536373

[10] Haber F, Weiss J. Über die Katalyse des hydroperoxydes (on the catalysis of hydroperoxide). Die Naturwissenschaften. 1932;**20**(51): 948-950. DOI: 10.1007/BF01504715

[11] Bedard K, Krause KH. The NOX family of ROS-generating NADPH oxidases: Physiology and pathophysiology. Physiological Reviews. 2007;**87**:245-313

[12] Bhattacharyya A, Chattopadhyay R, Mitra S, Crowe SE. Oxidative stress as an essential factor in the pathogenesis of gastrointestinal mucosal diseases. Physiological Reviews. 2014;**94**:329-354. DOI: 10.1152/physrev.00040.2012

[13] Ibrahim CB, Aroniadis OC, Brandt LJ. On the role of ischemia in the pathogenesis of IBD: A review. Inflammatory Bowel Diseases. 2010;**16**:696-702

[14] Baud L, Ardaillou R. Involvement of reactive oxygen species in kidney damage. British Medical Bulletin. 1993;**49**:62-629

[15] Forbes JM, Coughlan MT, Cooper ME. Oxidative stress as a major culprit in kidney disease in diabetes. Diabetes. 2008;**57**:1446-1454

[16] Colgan SP, Taylor CT. Hypoxia: An alarm signal during intestinal inflammation. Nature Reviews. Gastroenterology & Hepatology. 2010;**7**:281-287

[17] Iuchi T, Akaike M, Mitsui T, Ohshima Y, Shintani Y, Azuma H, et al. Glucocorticoid excess induces superoxide production in vascular endothelial cells and elicits vascular

endothelial dysfunction. Circulation Research. 2003;**92**:81-87

[18] Faraci FM. Oxidative stress: The curse that underlies cerebral vascular dysfunction? Stroke. 2005;**36**:186-188

[19] Butterfield DA, Reed TT, Perluigi M, De MC, Coccia R, Keller JN, et al. Elevated levels of 3-nitrotyrosine in brain from subjects with amnestic mild cognitive impairment: Implications for the role of nitration in the progression of Alzheimer's disease. Brain Research. 2007;**1148**:243-248

[20] Hamel E, Nicolakakis N, Aboulkassim T, Ongali B, Tong XK. Oxidative stress and cerebrovascular dysfunction in mouse models of Alzheimer's disease. Experimental Physiology. 2008;**93**:116-120

[21] Vandermosten L, Pham T-T, Possemiers H, Knoops S, Van Herck E, Deckers J, et al. Experimental malaria-associated acute respiratory distress syndrome is dependent on the parasite-host combination and coincides with normocyte invasion. Malaria Journal. 2018;**17**:102. DOI: 10.1186/s12936-018-2251-3

[22] Kerlin DH, Gatton ML. Preferential invasion by *Plasmodium* merozoites and the self-regulation of parasite burden. PLoS One. 2013;**8**:e57434

[23] Mavondo GA. Malaria disease perspective and an opinion: Should malaria treatment target the parasite or the malarial pathophysiology generated by the parasite or both? EC Microbiology. 2017;**7**(5):149-154

[24] Markus MB. Malaria: Origin of the term "hypnozoite". Journal of the History of Biology. 2011;**44**(4):781-786. DOI: 10.1007/s10739-010-9239-3

[25] Markus MB. Do hypnozoites cause relapse in malaria? Trends in Parasitology. 2015;**31**(6):239-245. DOI: 10.1016/j.pt.2015.02.003

[26] Mavondo GA, Mkhwananzi BN, Mabandla MV, Musabayane CT. Asiatic acid influences parasitaemia reduction and ameliorates malaria anaemia in *P. berghei* infected Sprague-Dawley male rats. BMC Complementary and Alternative Medicine. 2016;**16**(1):357. DOI: 10.1186/s12906-016-1338-z

[27] Buffet PA, Safeukui I, Deplaine G, Brousse V, Prendki V, Thellier M, et al. The pathogenesis of *Plasmodium falciparum* malaria in humans: Insights into splenic physiology. Blood. 2011;**117**(2):381-392. DOI: 10.1182/blood-2010-04-202911

[28] Khan R, Quaiser S, Haque SF. Malarial acute kidney injury: Prognostic markers. Annals of Tropical Medicine and Public Health. 2013;**6**:280-284

[29] Onwuamaegbu ME, Henein M, Coats AJ. Cachexia in malaria and heart failure: Therapeutic considerations in clinical practice. Postgraduate Medical Journal. 2004;**80**:642-649

[30] Mavondo GA, Mkhwananzi BN, Mabandla MV, Musabayane CT. Asiatic acid influences glucose homeostasis in *P. berghei* murine malaria infected Sprague Dawley rats. African Journal of Traditional, Complementary, and Alternative Medicines. 2016;**13**(5):91-101. DOI: 10.21010/ajtcam.v13i5.13

[31] White NJ, Warrell DA, Chanthanavich P, Looareesuwan S, Warrell MJ, Krishna S. Severe hypoglycaemia and hyperinsulinaemia in *falciparum* malaria. The New England Journal of Medicine. 1983;**309**:61-62

[32] Van den Steen PE, Deroost K, Deckers J, Van Herck E, Struyf S, Opdenakker G. Pathogenesis of malaria-associated acute respiratory distress

syndrome. Trends in Parasitology. 2013;**29**:346-358

[33] Mohan A, Sharma SK, Bollinen i S. Acute lung injury and acute respiratory distress syndrome in malaria. Journal of Vector Borne Diseases. 2008;**45**: 179-193

[34] Lin J, Sodenkamp J, Cunningham D, Deroost K, Tshitenge TC, McLaughlin S. Signatures of malaria-associated pathology revealed by highresolution whole-blood transcriptomics in a rodent model of malaria. Scientific Reports. 2017;7:41722

[35] Kateera F, Ingabire CH, Hakizimana E, Kalinda P, Mens PF, Grobusch MP. Malaria, anaemia and under-nutrition: Three frequently co-existing conditions among preschool children in rural Rwanda. Malaria Journal. 2015;**14**:440

[36] Thien H, Kager P, Sauerwein H. Hypoglycemia in falciparum malaria: Is fasting an unrecognized and insufficiently emphasized risk factor. Trends in Parasitology. 2006;**22**:410-415

[37] Mishra SK, Mahanta KC, Mohanty S. Malaria associated acute renal failure-experience from Rourkela, eastern India. Journal of the Indian Medical Association. 2008;**106**:640-654

[38] Day NP, Phu NH, Mai NT, Chau TT, Loc PP. The pathophysiologic and prognostic significance of acidosis in severe adult malaria. Critical Care Medicine. **28**:1833-1840

[39] Sharma L, Shukla G. Placental malaria: A new insight into the pathophysiology. Frontiers in Medicine. 2017;**4**:117. DOI: 10.3389/fmed.2017.00117

[40] Klayman DL. Qinghaosu (artemisinin): An antimalarial drug from China. Science. 1985;**228**:1049-1055

[41] Antoine T, Fisher N, Amewu R, O'Neill PM, Ward SA, Biagini GA. Rapid kill of malaria parasites by artemisinin and semi-synthetic endoperoxides involves ROS-dependent depolarization of the membrane potential. The Journal of Antimicrobial Chemotherapy. 2013;**69**(4):1005-1016. DOI: 10.1093/jac/dkt486

[42] Cui L, Su X-Z. Discovery, mechanisms of action and combination therapy of artemisinin. Expert Review of Anti-infective Therapy. 2009;**7**(8):999-1013. DOI: 10.1586/eri.09.68

[43] O'Neill PM, Barton VE, Ward SA. The molecular mechanism of action of artemisinin-the debate continues. Molecules. 2010;**15**:1705-1721

[44] Meshnick SR, Yang YZ, Lima V. Iron-dependent free radical generation from the antimalarial agent artemisinin (qinghaosu). Antimicrobial Agents and Chemotherapy. 1993;**37**:1108-1114

[45] Meshnick SR, Thomas A, Ranz A. Artemisinin (qinghaosu): The role of intracellular hemin in its mechanism of antimalarial action. Molecular and Biochemical Parasitology. 1991;**49**:181-189

[46] Posner GH, Oh CH, Wang D. Mechanism-based design, synthesis, and in vitro antimalarial testing of new 4-methylated trioxanes structurally related to artemisinin: The importance of a carbon-centered radical for antimalarial activity. Journal of Medicinal Chemistry. 1994;**37**:1256-1258

[47] Posner GH, Wang D, Cumming JN. Further evidence supporting the importance of and the restrictions on a carbon-centered radical for high antimalarial activity of 1,2,4-trioxanes like artemisinin. Journal of Medicinal Chemistry. 1995;**38**:2273-2275

[48] Butler AR, Gilbert BC, Hulme P. EPR evidence for the involvement of free radicals in the iron-catalysed decomposition of qinghaosu (artemisinin) and some derivatives; antimalarial action of some polycyclic endoperoxides. Free Radical Research. 1998;**28**:471-476

[49] Wu W-M, Wu Y, Y-L W. Unified mechanistic framework for the Fe(II)-induced cleavage of qinghaosu and derivatives/analogues. The first spin-trapping evidence for the previously postulated secondary C-4 radical. Journal of the American Chemical Society. 1998;**120**:3316-3325

[50] Robert A, Benoit-Vical F, Claparols C, Meunier B. The antimalarial drug artemisinin alkylates heme in infected mice. Proceedings of the National Academy of Sciences of the United States of America. 2005;**102**(38):13676-13680

[51] Wu Y. How might qinghaosu (artemisinin) and related compounds kill the intraerythrocytic malaria parasite? a chemist's view. Accounts of Chemical Research. 2002;**35**:255-259

[52] Shi C, Li H, Yang Y, Hou L. Anti-inflammatory and immunoregulatory functions of artemisinin and its derivatives. Mediators of Inflammation. 2015;**2015**:7. DOI: 10.1155/2015/435713

[53] Zhou WL, Wu JM, Wu QL. A novel artemisinin derivative, 3-(12-beta-artemisininoxy) phenoxyl succinic acid (SM735), mediates immunosuppressive effects in vitro and in vivo. Acta Pharmacologica Sinica. 2005;**26**(11):1352-1358

[54] Wang J-X, Tang W, Zhou R. The new water-soluble artemisinin derivative SM905 ameliorates collagen-induced arthritis by suppression of inflammatory and Th17 responses. British Journal of Pharmacology. 2008;**153**(6):1303-1310

[55] Wang J-X, Tang W, Yang Z-S. Suppressive effect of a novel water-soluble artemisinin derivative SM905 on T cell activation and proliferation in vitro and in vivo. European Journal of Pharmacology. 2007;**564**(1-3):211-218

[56] Zhao YG, Wang Y, Guo Z. Dihydroartemisinin ameliorates inflammatory disease by its reciprocal effects on Th and regulatory T cell function via modulating the mammalian target of rapamycin pathway. Journal of Immunology. 2012;**189**(9):4417-4425

[57] Hou L-F, He S-J, Li X. Sm934 treated lupus-prone NZB×NZW F1 mice by enhancing macrophage interleukin-10 production and suppressing pathogenic T cell development. PLoS One. 2012;**7**(2):e32424

[58] Hou L-F, He S-J, Li X. Oral administration of artemisinin analog SM934 ameliorates lupus syndromes in MRL/lpr mice by inhibiting Th1 and Th17 cell responses. Arthritis and Rheumatism. 2011;**63**(8):2445-2455

[59] Vennerstrom JL, Arbe-Barnes S, Brun R. Identification of an antimalarial synthetic trioxolane drug development candidate. Nature. 2004;**430**(7002):900-904

[60] Mercer AE, Maggs JL, Sun X-M. Evidence for the involvement of carbon-centered radicals in the induction of apoptotic cell death by artemisinin compounds. The Journal of Biological Chemistry. 2007;**282**(13):9372-9382

[61] Golenser J, Waknine JH, Krugliak M, Hunt NH, Grau GE. Current perspectives on the mechanism of action of artemisinins. International Journal for Parasitology. 2006;**36**(14):1427-1441

[62] Alberola-Ila J, Takaki S, Kerner JD, Perlmutter RM. Differential signaling by

lymphocyte antigen receptors. Annual Review of Immunology. 1997;**15**:125-154

[63] Lea NC, Orr SJ, Stoeber K. Commitment point during G0 → G1 that controls entry into the cell cycle. Molecular and Cellular Biology. 2003;**23**(7):2351-2361

[64] Li Y. Qinghaosu (artemisinin): Chemistry and pharmacology. Acta Pharmacologica Sinica. 2012;**33**(9):1141-1146

[65] Wang J-X, Tang W, Shi L-P. Investigation of the immunosuppressive activity of artemether on T-cell activation and proliferation. British Journal of Pharmacology. 2007;**150**(5):652-661

[66] Yang Z-S, Wang J-X, Zhou Y, Zuo J-P, Li Y. Synthesis and immunosuppressive activity of new artemisinin derivatives. Part 2: 2-[12(beta or alpha)-dihydroartemisinoxymethyl(or 1′-ethyl)]phenoxyl propionic acids and esters. Bioorganic & Medicinal Chemistry. 2006;**14**(23):8043-8049

[67] Zhang J-X, Wang J-X, Zhang Y. Synthesis and immunosuppressive activity of new artemisinin derivatives containing polyethylene glycol group. Yaoxue Xuebao. 2006;**41**(1):65-70

[68] Hou L-F, He S-J, Wang J-X. SM934, a water-soluble derivative of arteminisin, exerts immunosuppressive functions in vitro and in vivo. International Immunopharmacology. 2009;**9**(13-14):1509-1517

[69] Noori S, Hassan ZM, Rezaei B, Rustaiyan A, Habibi Z, Fallahian F. Artemisinin can inhibit the calmodulin-mediated activation of phosphodiesterase in comparison with cyclosporin A. International Immunopharmacology. 2008;**8**(13-14):1744-1747

[70] Noori S, Hassan ZM, Taghikhani M, Rezaei B, Habibi Z. Dihydroartemisinin can inhibit calmodulin, calmodulin-dependent phosphodiesterase activity and stimulate cellular immune responses. International Immunopharmacology. 2010;**10**(2):213-217

[71] Wang J-X, Hou L-F, Yang Y, Tang W, Li Y, Zuo JP. SM905, an artemisinin derivative, inhibited NO and proinflammatory cytokine production by suppressing MAPK and NF-B pathways in RAW 264.7 macrophages. Acta Pharmacologica Sinica. 2009;**30**(10):1428-1435

[72] He Y, Fan J, Lin H. The anti-malaria agent artesunate inhibits expression of vascular endothelial growth factor and hypoxia-inducible factor-1alpha in human rheumatoid arthritis fibroblast-like synoviocyte. Rheumatology International. 2015;**31**(1):53-60

[73] Xu H, He Y, Yang X. Anti-malarial agent artesunate inhibits TNF-alpha-induced production of proinflammatory cytokines via inhibition of NF-kB and PI3 kinase/Akt signal pathway in human rheumatoid arthritis fibroblast-like synoviocytes. Rheumatology. 2007;**46**(6):920-926

[74] Olliaro PL, Haynes RK, Meunier B, Yuthavong Y. Possible modes of action of the artemisinin-type compounds. Trends in Parasitology. 2001;**17**(3):122-126

[75] Eckstein-Ludwig U, Webb RJ, van Goethem IDA. Artemisinins target the SERCA of *Plasmodium falciparum*. Nature. 2003;**424**(6951):957-961

[76] Uhlemann A-C, Cameron A, Eckstein-Ludwig U. A single amino acid residue can determine the sensitivity of SERCAs to artemisinins. Nature Structural & Molecular Biology. 2005;**12**(7):628-629

[77] Jung M, Kim H, Ki YN, Kyoung TN. Three dimensional structure of *Plasmodium falciparum* Ca^{2+}-ATPase(PfATP6) and docking of artemisinin derivatives to PfATP6. Bioorganic & Medicinal Chemistry Letters. 2005;**15**(12):2994-2997

[78] Lv J, Sharma A, Zhang T, Wu Y, Ding X. Pharmacological review on asiatic acid and its derivatives: A potential compound. SLAS Technology. 2018;**23**(2):111-127. DOI: 10.1177/2472630317751840

[79] Mavondo GA, Musabayane CT. Asiatic acid-pectin hydrogel matrix patch transdermal delivery system influences parasitaemia suppression and inflammation reduction in *P. berghei* murine malaria infected Sprague-Dawley rats. Asian Pacific Journal of Tropical Medicine. 2016;**9**(12):1172-1180. DOI: 10.1016/j.apjtm.2016.10.008

[80] Mavondo GA, Musabayane CT. Transdermal drug delivery of asiatic acid influences renal function and electrolyte handling in *Plasmodium berghe*i-infected Sprague-Dawley male rats. Journal of Diseases and Medicinal Plants. 2018;**4**(1):18-29. DOI: 10.11648/j.jdmp.20180401.13

[81] Mavondo GA, Kasvosve I. Antimalarial phytochemicals: Delineation of the triterpene asiatic acid malarial anti-disease and pathophysiological remedial activities—Part I. Journal of Infectious Disease and Pathology. 2017;**1**:104

[82] Mavondo GA, Kasvosve I. Antimalarial phytochemicals: Delineation of the triterpene asiatic acid malarial anti-disease and pathophysiological remedial activities—Part II. Journal of Infectious Disease and Pathology. 2017;**1**:103

[83] Haldar K, Mohandas N. Malaria, erythrocytic infection and anemia. Hematology. American Society of Hematology. Education Program. 2009;**1**:87-93

[84] Skorokhod OA, Caione L, Marrocco T, Migliardi G, Barrera V, Arese P, et al. Inhibition of erythropoiesis in malaria anemia: Role of hemozoin and hemozoin-generated 4-hydroxynonenal. Blood. 2010;**116**(20):4328-4337. DOI: 10.1182/blood-2010-03-272781

[85] Fisher JW. Erythropoietin: Physiology and pharmacology update. Experimental Biology and Medicine. 2003;**228**:1-14

[86] Wu H, Klingmuller U, Besmer P, Lodish HF. Interaction of the erythropoietin and stem-cell-factor receptors. Nature. 1995;**377**:242-246

[87] Bachmann S, LeHir M, Eckardt KU. Co-localization of erythropoietin mRNA and ecto-5′-nucleotidase immunoreactivity in peritubular cells of rat renal cortex indicates that fibroblasts produce erythropoietin. The Journal of Histochemistry and Cytochemistry. 1993;**41**:335-341

[88] Maxwell PH, Osmond MK, Pugh CW, Heryet A, Nicholls LG, Tan CC, et al. Identification of the renal erythropoietin-producing cells using transgenic mice. Kidney International. 1993;**44**:1149-1162

[89] Fisher JW, Koury S, Ducey T, Mendel S. Erythropoietin production by interstitial cells of hypoxic monkey kidneys. British Journal of Haematology. 1996;**95**:27-32

[90] Mavondo GA, Musabayane CT. Transdermal drug delivery of asiatic acid influences renal function and electrolyte handling in plasmodium berghei-infected sprague-dawley male Rats. Journal of Diseases and Medicinal Plants. 2018;**4**(1):18-29

[91] Ghosh K, Ghosh K. Pathogenesis of anemia in malaria: A concise review. Parasitology Research. 2007;**101**:1463-1469

[92] Perkins DJ, Were T, Davenport GC, Kempaiah P, Hittner JB, Ong'echa JM. Severe malarial anemia: Innate immunity and pathogenesis. International Journal of Biological Sciences. 2011;**7**:1427-1442

[93] McDevitt MM, Xie J, Shanmugasundaram G, Griffith J, Liu A, McDonald C, et al. A critical role for the host mediator macrophage migration inhibitory factor in the pathogenesis of malarial anaemia. The Journal of Experimental Medicine. 2006;**203**:1185-1196

[94] Pradhan P. Malarial anaemia and nitric oxide induced megaloblastic anaemia: A review on the causes of malarial anaemia. Journal of Vector Borne Diseases. 2009;**46**:100-108

[95] Chang KH, Tam M, Stevenson MM. Inappropriately low reticulocytosis in severe malarial anemia correlates with suppression in the development of late erythroid precursor. Blood. 2004;**103**:3727-3735

[96] Autino B, Corbett Y, Castelli F, Taramelli D. Pathogenesis of malaria in tissues and blood. Mediterranean Journal of Hematology and Infectious Diseases. 2012;**4**(1):e2012061. DOI: 10.4084/MJHID.2012.061

[97] Huang SS, Chiu CS, Chen HJ, Hou WC, Sheu MJ. Antinociceptive activities and the mechanisms of anti-inflammation of asiatic acid in mice. Evidence-Based Complementary and Alternative Medicine. 2011;**2011**:10. DOI: 10.1155/2011/895857

[98] Chen H, Hua X-M, Ze B-C, Wang B, Wei L. The anti-inflammatory effects of asiatic acid in lipopolysaccharide-stimulated human corneal epithelial cells. International Journal of Ophthalmology. 2017;**10**(2):179-185. DOI: 10.18240/ijo.2017.02.01

[99] Xiao W, Jiang W, Li K, Hu Y, Li S, Zhou L, et al. Protective effect of asiatic acid in an experimental cerulein-induced model of acute pancreatitis in mice. American Journal of Translational Research. 2017;**9**(8):3842-3852

[100] Nemeth E, Rivera S, Gabayan V, Keller C, Taudorf S, Pedersen BK, et al. IL-6 mediates hypoferremia of inflammation by inducing the synthesis of the iron regulatory hormone hepcidin. The Journal of Clinical Investigation. 2004;**113**(9):1271-1276. DOI: 10.1172/JCI200420945

[101] Laftah AH, Sharma N, Brookes MJ, McKie AT, Simpson RJ, Iqbal TH, et al. Tumour necrosis factor α causes hypoferraemia and reduced intestinal iron absorption in mice. The Biochemical Journal. 2006;**397**(1):61-67. DOI: 10.1042/BJ20060215

[102] Amre Nasr A, Allam G, Hamid O, Al-Ghamdi A. IFN-gamma and TNF associated with severe *falciparum* malaria infection in Saudi pregnant women. Malaria Journal. 2014;**13**:314. DOI: 10.1186/1475-2875-13-314

[103] Lamikanra AA, Merryweather-Clarke AT, Tipping AJ, Roberts DJ. Distinct mechanisms of inadequate erythropoiesis induced by tumor necrosis factor alpha or malarial pigment. PLoS One. 2015;**10**(4):e0127124. DOI: 10.1371/journal.pone.0127124

[104] Boeuf PS, Loizon S, Awandare GA, Tetteh JKA, Addae MM, Adjei GO, et al. Insights into deregulated TNF and IL-10 production in malaria: Implications for understanding severe malarial anaemia. Malaria Journal. 2012;**11**:253. DOI: 10.1186/1475-2875-11-253©

[105] Nussenblatt V, Mukasa G, Metzger A, Ndeezi G, Garrett E, Semba RD. Anemia and interleukin-10, tumor necrosis factor alpha, and erythropoietin levels among children with acute, uncomplicated *Plasmodium falciparum* malaria. Clinical and Diagnostic Laboratory Immunology. 2001;**8**(6):1164-1170. DOI: 10.1128/CDLI.8.6.1164-1170.2001

[106] Sibiya H, Musabayane CT, Mabandla MV. Transdermal delivery of oleanolic acid attenuates pro-inflammatory cytokine release and ameliorates anaemia in *P. berghei* malaria. Acta Tropica. 2017;**171**:24-29. DOI: 10.1016/j.actatropica.2017.03.005

[107] Ramachandran V, Saravanan R. Asiatic acid prevents lipid peroxidation and improves antioxidant status in rats with streptozotocin-induced diabetes. Journal of Functional Foods. 2013;**5**:1077-1087

[108] Nanami M, Ookawara T, Otaki Y, Ito K, Moriguchi R, Miyagawa K, et al. Tumor necrosis factor-α–induced iron sequestration and oxidative stress in human endothelial cells. Arteriosclerosis, Thrombosis, and Vascular Biology. 2005;**25**:2495-2501. DOI: 10.1161/01.ATV.0000190610.63878.20

[109] Nemeth E, Tuttle MS, Powelson J, Vaughn MB, Donovan A, Ward DM, et al. Hepcidin regulates cellular iron efflux by binding to ferroportin and inducing its internalization. Science. 2004;**306**(5704):2090-2093

[110] de Mast Q, Syafruddin D, Keijmel S, Riekerink TO, Deky O, Asih PB, et al. Increased serum hepcidin and alterations in blood iron parameters associated with asymptomatic *P. falciparum* and *P. vivax* malaria. Haematologica. 2010;**95**:1068-1074

[111] Zhang DL, Wu J, Shah BN, Greutélaers KC, Ghosh MC, Ollivierre H, et al. Erythrocytic ferroportin reduces intracellular iron accumulation, hemolysis, and malaria risk. Science. 2018;**359**(6383):1520-1523. DOI: 10.1126/science.aal2022

[112] Zhang D-L, Ghosh MC, Ollivierre H, Li Y, Rouault TA. Ferroportin deficiency in erythroid cells causes serum iron deficiency and promotes hemolysis due to oxidative stress. Blood. 2018, 2018;(4):842997. DOI: 10.1182/blood-2018-04-842997

[113] Gwamaka M, Kurtis JD, Sorensen BE, Holte S, Morrison R, Mutabingwa TK, et al. Iron deficiency protects against severe *plasmodium falciparum* malaria and death in young children. Clinical Infectious Diseases. 2012;**54**(8):1137-1144. DOI: 10.1093/cid/cis010

[114] Prasetyani MA, de Mast Q, Afeworki R, Kaisar MMM, Stefanie D, Sartono E, et al. Effect of a short course of iron polymaltose on acquisition of malarial parasitaemia in anaemic Indonesian schoolchildren: A randomized trial. Malaria Journal. 2017;**16**:50. DOI: 10.1186/s12936-017-1691-5

[115] Kabyemela ER, Fried M, Kurtis JD, Mutabingwa TK, Duffy PE. Decreased susceptibility to *Plasmodium falciparum* infection in pregnant women with iron deficiency. The Journal of Infectious Diseases. 2008;**198**:163-166

[116] Clark MA, Goheen MM, Fulford A, Prentice AM, Elnagheeb MA, Patel J, et al. Host iron status and iron supplementation mediate susceptibility to erythrocytic stage *Plasmodium falciparum*. Nature Communications. 2014;**5**:4446. DOI: 10.1038/ncomms5446

[117] Zhang DL, Ghosh MC, Rouault TA. The physiological functions of iron regulatory proteins in iron homeostasis—An update. Frontiers

in Pharmacology. 2014;**5**:124. DOI: 10.3389/fphar.2014.00124

[118] Kasvosve I, Gomo ZAR, Nathoo KJ, Matibe P, Mudenge B, Loyevsky M, et al. Effect of ferroportin Q248H polymorphism on iron status in African children. The American Journal of Clinical Nutrition. 2005;**82**:1102-1106

[119] Gordeuk VR, Caleffi A, Corradini E, Ferrara F, Jones RA, Castro O, et al. Iron overload in Africans and African-Americans and a common mutation in the SCL40A1 (ferroportin 1) gene. Blood Cells, Molecules & Diseases. 2003;**31**(3):299-304

[120] Nekhai S, Xu M, Foster A, Kasvosve I, Diaz S, Machado RF, et al. Reduced sensitivity of the ferroportin Q248H mutant to physiological concentrations of hepcidin. Haematologica. 2013;**98**(3):455-463. DOI: 10.3324/haematol.2012.066530

[121] Zhang DL, Hughes RM, Ollivierre-Wilson H, Ghosh MC, Rouault TA. A ferroportin transcript that lacks an iron-responsive element enables duodenal and erythroid precursor cells to evade translational repression. Cell Metabolism. 2009;**9**(5):461-473. DOI: 10.1016/j.cmet.2009.03.006

[122] Zhang D-L, Senecal T, Ghosh MC, Ollivierre-Wilson H, Tu T, Rouault TA. Hepcidin regulates ferroportin expression and intracellular iron homeostasis of erythroblasts. Blood. 2011;**118**:2868-2877. DOI: 10.1182/blood-2011-01-330241

[123] Gonzales R, Auclair C, Voisin E, Gautero H, Dhermy D, Boivin P. Superoxide dismutase, catalase, and glutathione peroxidase in red blood cells from patients with malignant diseases. Cancer Research. 1984;**44**:4137-4139

[124] Nagababu E, Chrest FJ, Rifkind JM. Hydrogen-peroxide-induced heme degradation in red blood cells: The protective roles of catalase and glutathione peroxidase. Biochimica et Biophysica Acta. 2003;**1620**:211-217. DOI: 10.1016/S0304-4165(02)00537-8

[125] Nagababu E, Mohanty JG, Friedman JS, Rifkind JM. Role of peroxiredoxin-2 in protecting RBCs from hydrogen peroxide-induced oxidative stress. Free Radical Research. 2013;**47**:164-171. DOI: 10.3109/10715762.2012.756138

[126] Lee TH, Kim SU, Yu SL, Kim SH, Park DS, Moon HB. Peroxiredoxin II is essential for sustaining life span of erythrocytes in mice. Blood. 2003;**101**:5033-5038. DOI: 10.1182/blood-2002-08-2548

[127] Nagababu E, Mohanty JG, Bhamidipaty S, Ostera GR, Rifkind JM. Role of the membrane in the formation of heme degradation products in red blood cells. Life Sciences. 2010;**86**:133-138. DOI: 10.1016/j.lfs.2009.11.015

[128] Mohanty JG, Nagababu E, Rifkind JM. Red blood cell oxidative stress impairs oxygen delivery and induces red blood cell aging. Frontiers in Physiology. 2014;**5**:84. DOI: 10.3389/fphys.2014.00084

[129] Balagopalakrishna C, Manoharan PT, Abugo OO, Rifkind JM. Production of superoxide from hemoglobin-bound oxygen under hypoxic conditions. Biochemistry. 1996;**35**:6393-6398. DOI: 10.1021/bi952875+

[130] Abugo OO, Rifkind JM. Oxidation of hemoglobin and the enhancement produced by nitroblue tetrazolium. The Journal of Biological Chemistry. 1994;**269**:24845-24853

[131] Nagababu E, Gulyani S, Earley CJ, Cutler RG, Mattson MP, Rifkind JM. Iron-deficiency anaemia enhances red blood cell oxidative stress. Free Radical Research. 2008;**42**:824-829. DOI: 10.1080/10715760802459879

[132] Kiefmann R, Rifkind JM, Nagababu E, Bhattacharya J. Red blood cells induce hypoxic lung inflammation. Blood. 2008;**111**:5205-5214. DOI: 10.1182/blood-2007-09-113902

[133] Huertas A, Das SR, Emin M, Sun L, Rifkind JM, Bhattacharya J. Erythrocytes induce proinflammatory endothelial activation in hypoxia. American Journal of Respiratory Cell and Molecular Biology. 2013;**48**:78-86. DOI: 10.1165/rcmb.2011-0402OC

[134] George A, Pushkaran S, Konstantinidis DG, Koochaki S, Malik P, Mohandas N. Erythrocyte NADPH oxidase activity modulated by Rac GTPases, PKC, and plasma cytokines contributes to oxidative stress in sickle cell disease. Blood. 2013;**121**:2099-2107. DOI: 10.1182/blood-2012-07-441188

[135] Clementi ME, Giardina B, Colucci D, Galtieri A, Misiti F. Amyloid-beta peptide affects the oxygen dependence of erythrocyte metabolism: A role for caspase 3. The International Journal of Biochemistry & Cell Biology. 2007;**39**:727-735. DOI: 10.1016/j.biocel.2006.11.013

[136] Mandal D, Baudin-Creuza V, Bhattacharyya A, Pathak S, Delaunay J, Kundu M. Caspase 3-mediated proteolysis of the N-terminal cytoplasmic domain of the human erythroid anion exchanger 1 (band 3). The Journal of Biological Chemistry. 2003;**278**:52551-52558. DOI: 10.1074/jbc.M306914200

[137] Mandal D, Mazumder A, Das P, Kundu M, Basu J. Fas-, caspase 8-, and caspase 3-dependent signaling regulates the activity of the aminophospholipid translocase and phosphatidylserine externalization in human erythrocytes. The Journal of Biological Chemistry. 2005;**280**:39460-39467. DOI: 10.1074/jbc.M506928200

[138] Fens MH, van WR, Andringa G, van Rooijen KL, Dijstelbloem HM, Rasmussen JT. A role for activated endothelial cells in red blood cell clearance: Implications for vasopathology. Haematologica. 2012;**97**:500-508. DOI: 10.3324/haematol.2011.048694

[139] Kiefer CR, Snyder LM. Oxidation and erythrocyte senescence. Current Opinion in Hematology. 2000;**7**:113-116. DOI: 10.1097/00062752-200003000-00007

[140] Samaja M, Rubinacci A, Motterlini R, De PA, Portinaro N. Red cell aging and active calcium transport. Experimental Gerontology. 1990;**25**:279-286. DOI: 10.1016/0531-5565(90)90063-8

[141] Barodka V, Mohanty JG, Mustafa AK, Santhanam L, Nyhan A, Bhunia AK. Nitroprusside inhibits calcium-induced impairment of red blood cell deformability. Transfusion. 2013;**54**:434-444. DOI: 10.1111/trf.12291

[142] Jakeman GN, Saul A, Hogarth WL, Collins WE. Anaemia of acute malaria infections in non-immune patients primarily results from destruction of uninfected erythrocytes. Parasitology. 1999;**119**:127-133

[143] Weiss L. The red pulp of the spleen: Structural basis of blood flow. Clinics in Haematology. 1983;**12**:375-393

[144] Wang S, Dale GL, Song P, Viollet B, Zou MH. AMPKalpha1 deletion shortens erythrocyte life span in mice: Role of oxidative stress. The Journal of Biological Chemistry. 2010;**285**:19976-19985. DOI: 10.1074/jbc.M110.102467

[145] Mavondo GA, Mzingwane MML. Parasitic causes of hemolytic anemia: Severe malaria anemia pathophysiology, current and experiemental phytotherapeutics in malaria anemia. In: Khan J, editor. Current Topics on Anaemia. Rijeka, Croatia-EU: Intechopen; 2017

[146] Miller LH, Ackerman HC, X-z S, Wellems TE. Malaria biology and disease pathogenesis: Insights for new treatments. Nature Medicine. 2013;**19**(2):156-167

[147] Guzman NJ, Fang MZ, Tang SS, Ingelfinger JR, Garg LC. Autocrine inhibition of Na^+/K^+-ATPase by nitric oxide in mouse proximal tubule epithelial cells. The Journal of Clinical Investigation. 1995;**95**:2083-2088

[148] Roczniak A, Burns KD. Nitric oxide stimulates guanylate cyclase and regulates sodium transport in rabbit proximal tubule. The American Journal of Physiology. 1996;**270**:F106-F115

[149] Wambach G, Overhoff U, Hossmann V. Sodium transport and red cell deformability. Klinische Wochenschrift. 1985;**3**(Suppl. 3):35-37

[150] Rohn TT, Hinds TR, Vincenzi FF. Inhibition of Ca^{2+}-pump ATPase and the Na^+/K^+-pump ATPase by iron-generated free radicals. Protection by 6,7-dimethyl-2,4-DI-1-pyrrolidinyl-7H-pyrrolo[2,3-d] pyrimidine sulfate (U-89843D), a potent, novel, antioxidant/free radical scavenger. Biochemical Pharmacology. 1996;**51**:471-476

[151] Rohn TT, Hinds TR, Vincenzi FF. Ion transport ATPases as targets for free radical damage. Protection by an aminosteroid of the Ca^{2+} pump ATPase and Na^+/K^+ pump ATPase of human red blood cell membranes. Biochemical Pharmacology. 1993;**46**:525-534

[152] Clark IA, Cowden WB. The pathophysiology of *falciparum* malaria. Pharmacology & Therapeutics. 2003;**99**:221-260

[153] Zhang X, Wu J, Dou Y, Xia B, Rong W, Rimbach G, et al. Asiatic acid protects primary neurons against C-ceramide-induced apoptosis. European Journal of Pharmacology. 2012;**679**:51-59

[154] Asamoah KA, Robb DA, Furman BL. Chronic chloroquine treatment enhances insulin release in rats. Diabetes Research and Clinical Practice. 1990;**9**:273-278

[155] Phillips RE. Hypoglycaemia is an important complication of *falciparum* malaria. The Quarterly Journal of Medicine. 1989;**71**:477-483

[156] Mehta M, Sonawat HM, Sharma S. Malaria parasite-infected erythrocytes inhibit glucose utilization in uninfected red cells. FEBS Letters. 2005;**579**(27):6151-6158

[157] Krishna S, Waller DW, Terkuile F, Kwiatkowski D, Crawley J, Craddock CFC, et al. Lactic acidosis and hypoglycaemia in children with severe malaria-pathophysiological and prognostic significance. Transactions of the Royal Society of Tropical Medicine and Hygiene. 1994;**88**:67-73

[158] Warrell DA, Veall N, Chanthanavich P, Karbwang J, White NJ, Looareesuwan S, et al. Cerebral anaerobic glycolysis and reduced cerebral oxygen transport in human malaria. Lancet. 1988;**ii**:534-538

[159] English M, Sauerwein R, Waruiru C, Mosobo M, Obiero J, Lowe B, et al. Acidosis in severe childhood malaria. The Quarterly Journal of Medicine. 1997;**90**:263-270

[160] Melillo G, Musso T, Sica A, Taylor LS, Cox GW, Varesio L. A hypoxia-responsive element mediates a novel

pathway of activation of the inducible nitric oxide synthase promoter. The Journal of Experimental Medicine. 1995;**182**:1683-1693

[161] Baker RG, Hayden MS. NF-kB, infammation, and metabolic disease. Cell Metabolism. 2011;**15**:11-22

[162] Kettelhut I, Fiers W, Goldberg AL. The toxic effects of tumor necrosis factor in vivo and their prevention by cyclooxygenase inhibitors. Proceedings of the National Academy of Sciences of the United States of America. 1987;**84**:4273-4277

[163] Tracey KJ, Beutler B, Lowry SF, Merryweather J, Wolpe S, Milsark IW, et al. Shock and tissue injury induced by recombinant human cachectin. Science. 1986;**234**:470-474

[164] Grau GE, Fajardo LF, Piquet P-F, Allet B, Lambert P-H. Tumor necrosis factor (cachectin) as an essential mediator in murine cerebral malaria. Science. 1987;**237**:1210-1212

[165] Coxon RE, Fekade D, Knox K, Hussein K, Melka A. The efect of antibody against TNF alpha on cytokine response in Jarisch-Herxheimer reactions of louse-borne relapsing fever. The Quarterly Journal of Medicine. 1997;**90**:213-221

[166] Jesus JA, Lago JHG, Laurenti MD, Yamamoto ES, Passero LFD. Antimicrobial activity of oleanolic and ursolic acids: An update. Evidence-based Complementary and Alternative Medicine. 2015;**2015**:14. DOI: 10.1155/2015/620472

[167] Wen X, Sun H, Liu J, Cheng K, Zhang P, Zhang L, et al. Naturally occurring pentacyclic triterpenes as inhibitors of glycogen phosphorylase: Synthesis, structure-activity relationships, and X-ray crystallographic studies. Journal of Medicinal Chemistry. 2008;**51**:3540-3554

[168] Potz BA, Scrimgeour LA, Sabe SA, Clements RT, Sodha NR, Sellke FW. Glycogen synthase kinase 3β inhibition reduces mitochondrial oxidative stress in chronic myocardial ischemia. Journal of Thoracic and Cardiovascular Surgery. 2018;**155**(6):2492-2503. DOI: 10.1016/j.jtcvs.2017.12.127

[169] Elbadawi NEE, Mohamed MI, Dawod OY, Ali KE, Daoud OH, Ali EM, et al. Effect of quinine therapy on plasma glucose and plasma insulin levels in pregnant women infected with *Plasmodium falciparum* malaria in Gezira state. Eastern Mediterranean Health Journal. 2011;**17**:697-700

[170] Musabayane CT, Murambirwa P, Joosab N, Masola B, Mukaratirwa S. The effects of chloroquine on blood glucose and plasma insulin concentrations in male Sprague Dawley rats. Endocrine Abstracts. 2010;**21**:139

[171] Acquah S, Boampong JN, Eghan Jnr BA, Eriksson M. Evidence of insulin resistance in adult uncomplicated malaria: Result of a 2-year prospective study. Malaria Research and Treatment. 2014;**2014**:136148. DOI: 10.1155/2014/136148

[172] Ramachandran V, Saravanan R. Efcacy of asiatic acid, a pentacyclic triterpene on attenuating the key enzymes activities of carbohydrate metabolism in streptozotoc ininduced diabetic rats. Phytomedicine. 2013;**20**:230-236

[173] Schulman JL, Carleton JL, Whitney G, Whitehorn JC. Effect of glucagon on food intake and body weight in man. Journal of Applied Physiology. 1957;**11**:419-421

[174] Dabadghao VS, Singh VB, Sharma D, Meena BL. A study of serum lactate level in malaria and its correlation with severity of disease. International Journal

of Advanced Medical and Health Research. 2015;**2**:28-32

[175] Barsoum RS. Malarial aute renal failure. Journal of the American Society of Nephrology. 2000;**11**:2147-2154

[176] Dondorp AM, Day NP. The treatment of severe malaria. Transactions of the Royal Society of Tropical Medicine and Hygiene. 2007;**101**(7):633-634

[177] Thanachartwet V, Desakorn V, Sahassananda D, Win KKYK, Supaporn T. Acute renal failure in patients with severe *falciparum* malaria: Using the WHO 2006 and RIFLE criteria. International Journal of Nephrology. 2013;**2013**:6. DOI: 10.1155/2013/841518

[178] Raffray L, Receveur M-C, Beguet M, Lauroua P, Pistone T, Malvy D. Severe delayed autoimmune haemolytic anaemia following artesunate administration in severe malaria: A case report. Malaria Journal. 2014;**13**:398. Available from: http://www.malariajournal.com/content/13/1/398

[179] Percário S, Moreira DR, Gomes BAQ, Ferreira MES, Gonçalves ACM, Laurindo PSO, et al. Oxidative stress in malaria. International Journal of Molecular Sciences. 2012;**13**(12): 16346-16372. DOI: 10.3390/ijms131216346

[180] Maitland K, Pamba A, Fegan G, Njuguna P, Nadel S, Newton CRJC, et al. Perturbations in electrolyte levels in Kenyan children with severe malaria complicated by acidosis. Clinical Infectious Diseases. 2005;**40**(1):9-16. DOI: 10.1086/426022

[181] Hanson J, Hossain A, Charunwatthana P, Hassan MU, Davis TME, Lam SWK, et al. Hyponatremia in severe malaria: Evidence for an appropriate anti-diuretic hormone response to hypovolemia. The American Journal of Tropical Medicine and Hygiene. 2009;**80**(1):141-145

[182] Musabayane CT, Munjeri O, Matavire TP. Transdermal delivery of chloroquine by amidated pectin hydrogel matrix patch in the rat. Renal Failure. 2003;**25**(4):525-534

[183] Giovanella F, Ferreira GK, de Prá SDT, Carvalho-Silva M, Gomes LM, Scaini G, et al. Effects of primaquine and chloroquine on oxidative stress parameters in rats. Annals of the Brazilian Academy of Sciences. 2015;**87**(2):1487-1496. DOI: 10.1590/0001-3765201520140637

[184] Patel H, Dhangar K, Sonawane Y, Surana S, Karpoormath R, Thapliyal N, et al. In search of selective 11b-HSD type 1 inhibitors without nephrotoxicity: An approach to resolve the metabolic syndrome by virtual based screening. Arabian Journal of Chemistry. 2018;**11**:221-232. DOI: 10.1016/j.arabjc.2015.08.003

[185] Stewart PM, Worwood CB, Walker BR. Steroid hormones and hypertension: The cortisol-cortisone shuttle. Steroids. 1993;**58**:614-620

[186] Walker BR, Connacher AA, Lindsay RM, Webb DJ, Edwards CRW. Carbenoxolone increases hepatic insulin sensitivity in man: A novel role for 11-oxosteroid reductase in enhancing glucocorticoid receptor activation. The Journal of Clinical Endocrinology and Metabolism. 1995;**80**:3155-3159

[187] Kotelevtsev Y, Brown R, Fleming WS, Kenyon C, Edwards CRW, Seckl JR, et al. Hypertension inmice lacking 11b hydroxysteroid dehydrogenase type 2. The Journal of Clinical Investigation. 1999;**103**:683-689

[188] Park SB, Park JS, Jung WH, Kim HK, Kwak HJ, Ahn JH, et al.

Anti-inflammatory effect of a selective 11b-hydroxysteroid dehydrogenase type 1 inhibitor via the stimulation of heme oxygenase-1 in LPS-activated mice and J774.1 murine macrophages. Journal of Pharmacological Sciences. 2016;**131**: 241-250. DOI: 10.1016/j.jphs.2016.07.003

[189] Puigoriol-Illamola D, Griñán-Ferré C, Vasilopoulou F, Leiva R, Vázquez S, Pallàs M. 11β-HSD1 inhibition by RL-118 promotes autophagy and correlates with reduced oxidative stress and inflammation, enhancing cognitive performance in SAMP8 mouse model. Molecular Neurobiology. 2018;**55**(12):8904-8915. DOI: 10.1007/s12035-018-1026-8

Chapter 3

Plasmodium falciparum Protein Exported in Erythrocyte and Mechanism Resistance to Malaria

Neyder Contreras-Puentes

Abstract

Malaria is a tropical disease of parasitic origin transmitted by the Anopheles mosquito, caused by the protozoan of the genus *Plasmodium*. Around miles of people worldwide affected by disease, have been related the endemic development of genetic alterations, called erythrocyte polymorphisms. These erythrocyte polymorphisms have become tools for resistance against malaria, where they have had an impact on the appearance of hemoglobinopathies, enzymatic alterations in erythrocytes, and modifications in the structure of erythrocytes related to membrane proteins. These sections address a detailed approach to the resistance mechanisms involved against the development of *P. falciparum* and develop a complete development of the principles of molecular principles that attempt to explain the functioning of these biochemical mechanisms and the development of the parasite.

Keywords: malaria, *Plasmodium falciparum*, erythrocyte, polymorphism, protein, hemoglobinopathies

1. Introduction

Malaria is one of the world's most severe public health problems. It leads to high rates of morbidity and mortality in many underdeveloped countries, where children and pregnant women are the most affected groups. According to the World Malaria Report by the World Health Organization (WHO), 3.5 billion people from 106 countries live in areas where they are in risk of transmission, representing half of the world's population [1]. On the other hand, malaria caused an estimated 200 million clinical episodes and 445,000 deaths, 90% of these deaths in Africa [2, 3]. Malaria is caused by parasites of the *Plasmodium* genus, which are intracellular eukaryotic organisms, with a complex life cycle. They commute between an invertebrate transmitter vector, where the sexual stages develop, and a vertebrate host, where the asexual stages take place. *P. falciparum* is responsible for the severe forms of malaria and the majority of annual deaths [4, 5].

Human malaria clinical signs and symptoms are a direct consequence of the parasite's life cycle. Humans are infected with *P. falciparum* sporozoites, through the female Anopheles mosquito's bite. Each sporozoite reaches the liver through blood or lymphatic circulation and multiplies forming a liver schizont, which differentiates into thousands of merozoites that are released into the bloodstream, after the schizont ruptures. Once released into the systemic circulation, the merozoites invade

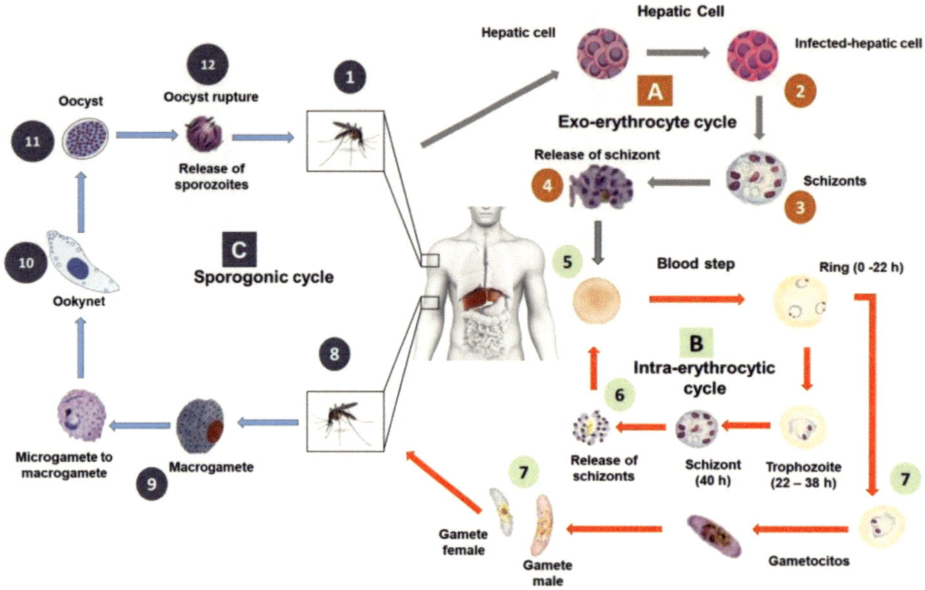

Figure 1.
Life cycle of Plasmodium spp. A. Exoerythrocytic cycle (1). Anopheles mosquito inoculates the sporozoites with subsequent invasion in liver cells (2); generation of first pre-erythrocytic schizogony (3). B. Erythrocytic cycle. The rupture of the schizont (4) releases the merozoites into the bloodstream where they invade red blood cells (5) forming a trophozoite that ripens into schizont, whose rupture releases merozoites back into the torrent (6). Some trophozoites can mature into gametocytes (7) that are ingested by the mosquito (8). C. Sporogonic cycle. The gametocytes mature to macrogametes and flagellated microgametes (9) that, after fertilization, produce an ooquineto (10), which migrates from the mosquito to generate oocyst (11) that will release thousands of sporozoites (12). Adapted from http://www.dpd.cdc.gov/dpdx/HTML/ImageLibrary/Malaria_il.htm.

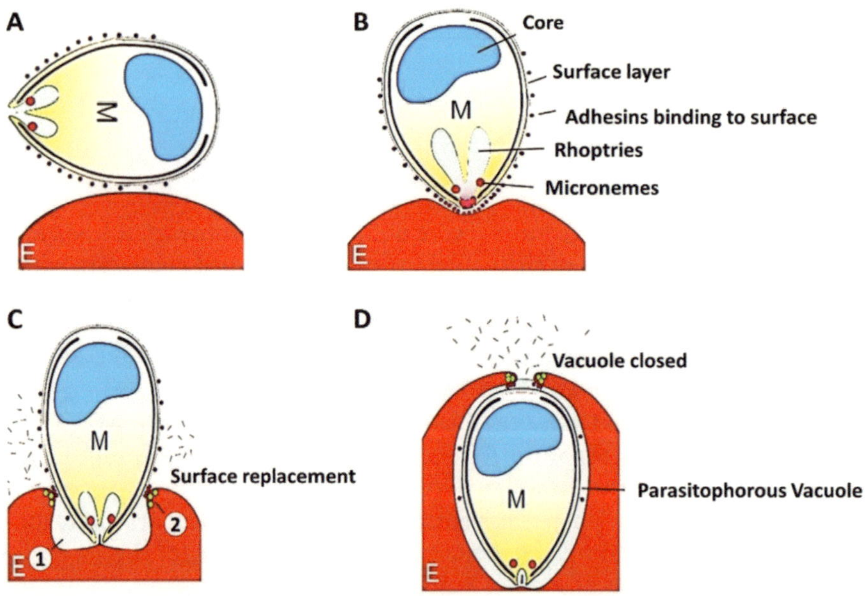

Figure 2.
Merozoite invasion process in human erythrocytes. Description of invasion and internalization of the P. falciparum parasite in the host cell. (1) The nascent parasitophorous vacuole. (2) Contact closed. (A) Initial contact of merozoite to erythrocyte. (B) The adhesion of the merozoite to the erythrocyte is observed, through the specific recognition and interaction of antigens and antibodies, as well as the functional and structural role of the micronemes and rhoptries. (C) Process of invasion and development of the parasitophorous vacuole. (D) The internalization of the merozoite in the new host cell and the complete formation of the parasitophorous vacuole are detailed. Taken and adapted from Zuccala and Baum [30].

the red blood cells and initiate the intra-erythrocyte stage, which lasts approximately 48 hours. Immediately after the invasion, the growth and development staging begins first as rings (0–24 h), then as trophozoites (24–40 h), and finally as schizonts (40–48 h); the cycle ends with the host cell destruction and the release of new merozoites from circulating erythrocytes, then initiating another cycle [6] (**Figure 1**).

During the development and growth stages, the parasite causes successive changes in the architecture of the infected erythrocyte (remodeling), which are fundamental for its vital functions. These changes are the acquisition of extracellular environment nutrients, the attribution of cytoadhesive properties that contribute to spleen-clearance evasion, the generation of changes in the host membrane cytoskeleton that are necessary for efficient parasite progeny release, and the formation of new organelles, such as the Maurer's clefts, tubulovesicular network, and the parasitophorous vacuole membrane (PVM) (**Figure 2**) [7, 8]. When the parasite enters the erythrocyte, it locates inside a parasitophorous vacuole (PV), which isolates it from the host cell cytoplasm, through the PVM. From then on, pathogen survival will depend on the efficient traffic of the molecules through the PVM and the plasma membrane [4, 9].

2. Human erythrocyte: properties of the human erythrocyte membrane

The erythrocyte is a cell of approximately 8 μm in diameter, highly specialized in O_2 and CO_2 transportation, without a nucleus and other organelles, useful for protein synthesis. It has the ability to transit the bloodstream over a 120-days lifetime. In addition, it has a remarkable capacity for deformability that allows its movement through the capillary microcirculation and splenic endothelial clefts in approximately 1 μm diameter [10]. The erythrocyte elastic properties are due to the cytoskeleton membrane, which is formed by an array of regular hexagonal proteins which makes up a two-dimensional mesh on the cell's cytoplasmic surface. These structural proteins interact with membrane lipids to maintain fluidity and subdivide them into three protein types: cytoskeleton, integral, and anchor [11].

The membrane cytoskeleton proteins underlie just under the lipid bilayer and associate with other proteins, forming a dynamic protein network, responsible for maintaining the integrity of the erythrocyte, as it passes through narrow blood capillaries. Spectrin, actin, adducin, dematin, band 4.1, tropomyosin, and tropomodulin are within this group. Integral proteins are characterized for being embedded in the lipid bilayer and presenting intra and extracellular domains, such

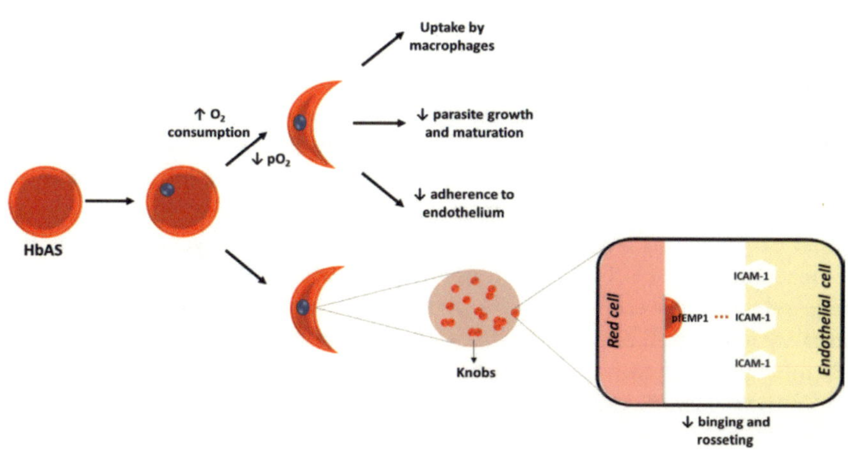

Figure 3.
Mechanisms of HbAS-related protection against P. falciparum. Adapted of Bunn [81].

as band 3 and glycophorin A and C. Finally, anchoring proteins have the function of connecting the cytoskeleton proteins with integral proteins, such as ankyrins and band 4.2 proteins [12, 13].

3. Erythrocyte and merozoite membrane proteins: participate in *P. falciparum* invasion process

The remodeling of the structures of the human erythrocytes for parasite of the malaria is generated between the process of invasion of merozoites. During the process, the parasite induces a transitory alteration of the structure of the membrane of the host cell, binging sites of the surface cellular [14]. More than 50 *P. falciparum* proteins have been identified which induce the process of invasion; however, some functional classes of elements such as merozoite surface protein (MSPs) have been described, which have demonstrated a structural complex around the envelope of the merozoites, related to PfEBAs (*P. falciparum* erythrocyte binding antigens) and PfRHs (*P. falciparum* reticulocytes binding protein), which are able of save organelles as micronemes and rhoptries [15–17].

In general, the erythrocyte membrane changes are set in motion with the merozoite invasion process. It has been described that the initial interaction between the merozoite and erythrocyte is probably a random collision, depending on the function of actin-myosin binding and specific molecular interactions between merozoite ligands and erythrocyte membrane receptors, which mediate cellular recognition and invasion of red blood cells [18]. This invasive process is carried out in four steps. The first step, called the initial contact with merozoite, takes place mainly by the interaction of proteins that are uniformly distributed on the surface of the merozoite, called glycosyl-phosphatidyl-inositol protein (GPI), with erythrocyte surface ligands, such as merozoite surface protein 1 (MSP1), whose receptor is band 3 protein in the erythrocyte membrane [19, 20]. The second step is called reorientation, which is produced for vertical arrangement of apical secretory organelles, such as rhoptries and micronemes. This step is mediated by a protein called apical membrane Antigen-1 (AMA1), which seems to establish the apical interaction of the adhesins with the erythrocyte; it is the border point between the weak union that occurs in the initial contact with MSP1 and irreversible bonds that occur between microneme proteins and erythrocyte membrane proteins [21, 22]. The third step is the tight-binding formation between various adhesins produced at the apical end of the parasite and its membrane receptors in the red blood cell, where the Duffy binding-like proteins (DBL) and reticulocyte binding proteins (RBP) bind. For example, surface DBL proteins of merozoite EBA 175 and EBA 140 (erythrocyte binding antigen 175 and 140) bind to erythrocyte membrane sialoglycoproteins, such as glycophorin A and C [23, 24]. On the other hand, while PfRh proteins bind to complement receptor 1 (CR1), signalization established by sensitive chymotrypsin receptor pathway and resistant to neuraminidase takes place [23, 25]. Once the parasite and erythrocyte tight junction is established, intake is mediated by the actin-myosin motor activation on the merozoite surface. This coincides with lipid and protein secretion, such as organelle-released proteases called rhoptries, micronemes, and mononemes. These proteases are associated to perform integral membrane proteins cleavage, such as band 3 and rupture of the membrane cytoskeletal proteins [26, 27].

During the invasion, proteins from the rhoptries and dense granules are secreted into the parasitophorous vacuole, and once it has developed to the ring phase, these proteins are exported to the cytoplasm of the infected erythrocyte to trigger the succession of effects of remodeling at the level of the host cell. It has been established that *P. falciparum* is capable of associating with Knobs, which are related to Knobs-proteins rich in histidines (KHARP). This type of formations allows the presentation of cytoadherence proteins exported by the parasite, which are coupled to the membrane, as is the case in particular of *P. falciparum* of erythrocyte membrane protein 1 (PfEMP1) [27].

Subsequently, the parasite invaginates the erythrocyte through a protein-free zone and initiates the formation of parasitophorous vacuole, which continues with a motility mechanism to enter the host cell. Rhoptries and dense granules secrete proteins during the invasion early ring phase, which are trafficked to different structures, such as parasitophorous vacuoles, cytosol, and erythrocyte membrane, triggering a series of events that modify the host cell [28].

4. *P. falciparum* export proteins modify the erythrocyte membrane.

Once inside the erythrocyte, *P. falciparum* is subjected to a trophic phase, followed by a replicative phase. The parasite modifies the host cell during the intra-erythrocytic period, conditioning it as its new habitat. It induces the formation of new permeability pathways, allowing it to provide itself with essential nutrients, dispose of waste products, modify the electrolytic composition, and decrease the colloid osmotic pressure of the erythrocyte, in order to survive in this new environment [29].

The infected erythrocyte enlarges in size, developing the formation of parasitophorous vacuole (PV), parasitophorous vacuole membrane (PVM), new membranous structures, such as the Maurer's clefts (MC), tubulovesicular networks (TVN), and erythrocyte surface protrusion appearance called Knobs. Moreover, new type of channels in the PVM and alterations of the erythrocytic membrane channels are formed, in which virulence proteins are trafficked [7, 29, 30]. In addition to MC and TVM, other structures have been described, which are involved in export protein trafficking, such as electron-dense vesicles (EDV), vesicle-like structures (VLS), J points or J-Dots, named for J-domain proteins [31–34].

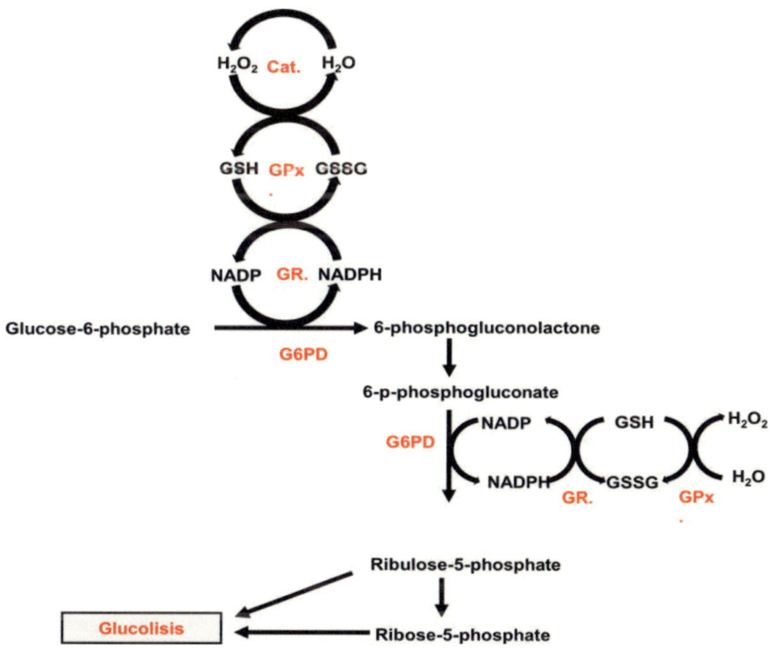

Figure 4.
Glucose-6-phosphate dehydrogenase (G6PD) pathway. G6PD, glucose-6-phosphate dehydrogenase, GPX, glutathione peroxidase; GR, glutathione reductase, 6PG, 6-phosphogluconate dehydrogenase; GSH, glutathione reduced; GSSG: glutathione oxidized. Adapted from Cappellini and Fiorelli [92].

Name of identification	Protein	Location	Molecular weight (kDa)	Putative function	References
KAHRP	Knob-associated histidine-rich protein	Erythrocyte cytoskeleton	85–105	Essential for the formation of Knobs; joins the erythrocyte spectrin, actin, and cytoplasmic tail of PfEMP-1	[40, 41]
MESA/PfEMP2	Mature parasite-infected erythrocyte surface antigen	Erythrocyte cytoskeleton	168	It binds to the protein 4.1R. You can interrupt the interaction p55–4.1R	[41–43]
RESA/PF155	Ring-infected erythrocyte surface antigen	Erythrocyte cytoskeleton	127	Joins the spectrin. Suppresses the increase of heat-induced membrane. It can stabilize the erythrocyte membrane. Could prevent the invasion of erythrocytes parasitized	[44–46]
Antigen 332 (Pf332)	*P. falciparum* antigen 332	Erythrocyte cytoskeleton and Maurer's clefts	700	Binds with the protein actin and provides deformability of erythrocytes	[47]
GBP130	Glycophorin binding protein 130	Erythrocyte cytoplasm and membrane of parasitophorous vacuole	105	Decrease of rigidity	[48]
PfEMP3	*P. falciparum* erythrocyte membrane protein 3	Erythrocyte cytoskeleton and Maurer's clefts	274–315	Joins the spectrin. Interrupts the interaction of the actin-spectrin-4.1R protein complex. Involved in the trafficking of PfEMP1.	[41, 49]
PfEMP1	*P. falciparum* erythrocyte membrane protein 1	Erythrocyte membrane and Maurer's clefts	200–250	Cytoadherence ligand, antigenic variation, and interacts with KARHP	[50]
RIFIN	Repetitive interspersed family	Maurer's Clefts and erythrocyte surface	—	Possibly antigenic variability	[38]
STEVOR	Subtelomeric variable open reading frame	Maurer's Clefts and erythrocyte surface	—	Possibly antigenic variability	[51]
SURFIN 4.2	Surface-associated interspersed gene protein 4.2	Maurer's Clefts and erythrocyte surface	—	Possibly antigenic variability	[52]

Name of identification	Protein	Location	Molecular weight (kDa)	Putative function	References
MAHRP1	Membrane-associated histidine-rich protein 1	Erythrocyte membrane	28.9	Generating the Maurer's clefts or in protecting proteins within these structures	[53]
REX-1	Ring-exported protein 1	Transmembrane	83	ND	[54]

ND, nondeterminate.

Table 1.
Proteins from the export of P. falciparum that modify post-invasion erythrocyte [6, 9].

Another host cell modification refers to *P. falciparum* infected erythrocyte cytoadherence to endothelial cells, resulting in a sequestration of mature parasites in capillaries and microvasculature [35]. The sequestration probably leads to microcirculation alterations and metabolic dysfunctions, which could be responsible for severe malaria manifestations [36]. The cytoadherence to endothelial cells confers at least two advantages for the parasite: (1) a more suitable microaerophilic environment for parasite metabolism and (2) evasion to splenic circulation, where infected erythrocytes would be destroyed [36–39]. *P. falciparum* exports its proteins to the erythrocyte cytoplasm, where it binds to cytoskeletal components and alters the natural interactions of the membrane structural proteins, in order to achieve these major changes in the erythrocyte structure. Export proteins are encoded by 8% of *P. falciparum* parasite genome. It corresponds to host cell exported proteins, both in asexual and gametophytic phases. **Table 1** lists the main *P. falciparum* export proteins, which participate in the remodeling process and present PEXEL motifs. However, non-PEXEL proteins such as PfEMP1, SURFIN, and Pf332 are also shown in **Table 1**, due to their importance in the infected erythrocyte remodeling process, but only PfEMP1.

5. Mechanism of resistance to malaria and effect of *P. falciparum* in erythrocyte

Parasites of the genus *Plasmodium* have co-evolved over 200 million years with the human species [55]. In this way, the increase of migrations in multiple regions and the establishment of settlements in certain areas have influenced the increase in endemicity produced by the successive exposure of the etiological agent of the disease; this high effect of selective pressure of the parasite has co-influenced the development of genetic variations linked to endemic populations, from which they have emerged over time polymorphic variants in erythrocytes in order to respond to the most severe symptoms of the disease, hindering the survival of the parasite or preventing the development of its entire life cycle. Many of these variations may be due to changes in structural proteins of the erythrocyte, alterations in hemoglobin (thalassemia's and sickle cell anemia), or an incidence in the quantitative and functional level of enzyme activity involved in oxidative processes such as G6PD or pyruvate kinase [56, 57].

Currently, a global distribution of erythrocyte polymorphisms has been described, such as hemoglobinopathies (thalassemia's, HbS, HbC, and HbE) and enzymatic alterations such as glucose-6-phosphate dehydrogenase deficiency (G6PD), which have their origin in response to the selective pressure exerted by malaria parasites on humans during the last 70,000 years [58]. Therefore, hemoglobinopathies and erythroenzymopathies have been attributed to different mechanisms that provide protection against severe manifestations of malaria; some of the relevant mechanisms are associated with reduced erythrocyte invasion, decreased intraerythrocytic growth, increased phagocytosis in infected erythrocytes, and increased immune response against parasitized erythrocytes [59]. Therefore, this type of erythrocyte polymorphisms can be related to resistance to malaria through immune mechanisms that can be a major health problem, due to the high frequency of carriers in endemic areas of malaria, mainly in the African continent where this It seriously affects the normal development of populations. Therefore, this type of genetic variants was originally characteristic of the tropics and subtropics; nowadays, there is a high dispersion in the whole world, product of the continuous migrations that induce an increased effect of the prevalence values of these diseases [60].

5.1 Hemoglobinopathies

Hemoglobinopathies are a group of genetic alterations that involve a change in some of the subunits of hemoglobin and present an autosomal recessive inheritance pattern [61, 62]. These are divided into structural hemoglobinopathies, produced by the simple substitution of amino acids in the α and β chains of hemoglobin and thalassemic syndromes, which are manifested by the total or partial decrease in the synthesis of a globin chain [63]. The frequency of these polymorphisms in the world population and their geographical distribution are highly variable. In the case of hemoglobinopathies, it is estimated that every year more than 300,000 children with severe forms of these diseases are born worldwide, most of them in countries of low and medium income [64, 65]. Approximately 5% of the world population carries a sickle cell or thalassemia gene, and in some regions, the percentage of carriers can reach 25%. Approximately 60–70% of all births of children with some serious alteration of hemoglobin (Hb) occurs in Africa, being the sub-Saharan region the most affected [66, 67].

5.1.1 Hemoglobin S

Hemoglobin S (HbS) is associated with a mutation in the β-globin gene where there is a change of thymine by adenine, thus coding a valine instead of glutamic acid (Glu6Val, βS). This mutation produces a hydrophobic modification in the deoxygenation of the Hb tetramer, which results in the union between the beta-1 and beta-2 chains of the two hemoglobin molecules (Hb). This union produces a polymer nucleus, which grows and invades erythrocytes, affecting architecture and flexibility and influencing cellular dehydration, with physical and oxidative cellular stress [68]. HbS is a hereditary trait that follows an autosomal recessive pattern, and therefore, it can present in a homozygous (HbSS) or heterozygous (HbAS) form. The HbSS form causes sickle cell anemia (SCA), while the heterozygote is considered a carrier of the trait [69].

It is estimated that around of 300 million people in the world, are diagnosed with sickle cell trait (SCT) a greater presence in Africa and the Mediterranean region, where the endemic areas of malaria are related to the occurrence of these hemoglobinopathies. In the United States, the prevalence of sickle cell traits is estimated at 8% for African-Americans and 0.05% for white Americans, suggesting an approximate incidence of 7.9 per 100,000 births. [70, 71].

At the metabolic level, it has been described that an increase in the production of ROS in the erythrocytes of individuals carrying the sickle trait shows a behavior similar to senescent erythrocytes. This phenomenon describes that aging causes erythrocyte cytosolic changes that affect antioxidant functioning, which can lead to the generation of a redox imbalance and induce the hemolysis and toxic accumulation of heme and Hb in the plasma [72, 73]. This oxidative imbalance tends to be even greater in the erythrocytes of carrier individuals, a process that increases in cytosolic and membrane transformations due to the decrease in its half-life. Hence, the infection of HbAS erythrocytes with malaria parasites causes an increase in the redox imbalance associated with the metabolic activity of the pathogens. However, the molecular effects of this imbalance are not fully established and therefore it is necessary to continue with their study to establish their role in the parasitic-host relationship.

Equally, have been suggested mechanisms which the sickle cell protects against malaria as shown by Pasvol et al., where an inhibition of growth of the parasite due to the polymerization of HbS and effect related with low oxygen levels is presented [74, 75]. Recently, Archer et al. demonstrated that infected erythrocytes HbAS showed a decrease in oxygen levels affecting the intracellular growth. These investigations have evidenced that growth inhibition produced by HbS-polymerized increments the cytoadherence, a condition favorable for inducing a reduction in the development of parasites [76].

Other mechanisms related have evidenced morphologic modifications in erythrocyte due to aberrant expression of PfEMP1 able of affect the binding of infected RBCs to host cells, and induce the diminution of virulence through the reduction of rosette formation and decreased cytoadherence [77]. Also, it has been described that the generation of antibodies against band-3 protein may be associated with formation of aggregated band-3 with impact in new sites for endothelium adhesion on erythrocyte with such polymorphisms and finally able cause conformational changes in band-3. Alike, it has been demonstrated that the parasite remodels the interaction of actin-cytoskeleton binding to enable the export of parasite-derived proteins to knobs on the parasitized RBC surface [58] **Figure 3**.

Thus, the mechanism established that during the invasive step in sickle cell, all are affected to a phenomenon of oxidative stress. This increase in ROS induces phagocytosis phenomenon related with hemoglobin denaturation, formation and hemichrome binding, aggregation protein as band 3 protein, development of antibody and it deposition, and binding of complement C3c fragments [78].

In this way, the increase of phagocytosis processes in HbAS erythrocytes infected with *P. falciparum* is remarkably advantageous for the host, in which a succession of associated mechanisms is triggered such as growth reduction and population density of parasites, young forms of the parasite are rapidly eliminated by the immune response, and it has been observed that mature forms (trophozoites and schizonts) adhere to the endothelium in smaller proportion in important organs (lungs, kidneys, brain, bone marrow, and placenta), which has led to a decrease in the severe symptoms of the disease (cerebral malaria, placental malaria, and respiratory disorders) [79, 80].

On the other hand, some molecular mechanisms have been established which have included the concept of microRNA (miRNAs). The development in cultures have founded the action of two miRNAs, miR-451 and let-7i, regulating of growth of parasites. Likewise, the incidence of miR-451 and let7i have induced reduction of parasitemia and a notable effect in the incorporation of hypoxanthine producing changes in characteristic of erythrocyte and defects during invasion of parasite, which have been associated with high specificity of sequences of miRNAs with anti-parasite function.

5.1.2 α- and β-thalassemia

During much time, the association between α-thalassemia and malarial protection mechanism has been studied, reporting the presence of the α + variety in the studied population [82]. The α-thalassemia is able to induce hemolytic state and be associated with a reduction in erythrocyte survival, with an increased erythrocyte in circulating young erythrocytes [83]. The α-thalassemia is very common in malaria-endemic regions; it is considered to confer protection against clinical manifestations of the disease induced by *P. falciparum*. *In vitro* studies have evidenced that in α-thalassemic erythrocytes infected with *Plasmodium*, high levels of antibodies develop from their surface. Additionally, activation mechanisms in opsonized erythrocytes, complement-induced lysis and inhibition of sequestration of infected erythrocytes have been associated, which result as anti-malarial mechanisms that might be promoted by such antibodies [84, 85].

In other studies, the roles of microcytosis have been associated with the protection from *P. falciparum*-related hemoglobin decrease; in patients, a reduction of infection for part of parasite and most notary in homozygous α-thalassemic individuals have been evidenced, where a decline of hemoglobin levels, is observed and likewise, microcytosis is related with oxidative stress induced in altered erythrocytes with the presence of thalassemia and iron-deficiency. Finally, could be linked a development of process as low resetting in infected microcytic RBCs [86]. Likewise, α-thalassemia protects against severe malaria by attenuating the effect of parasite virulence and decreasing the amount of Hb loss during increased parasitemia. The α-thalassemia erythrocytes parasitized may be more susceptible to phagocytosis in vitro culture and unavailable than normal red cells in the formation of rosettes [87, 88]. Alike, has been related the complement receptor 1 (CR1), which is reduced on α-thalassemic erythrocytes infected, the diminution of CR1 expression in this type of cells are associated with a possible mechanism for reduction resetting [89]. Following, with less able to adhere to endothelial cells. Of this mode, studies have suggested that altered cells maintain that membrane band 3 may be a target for enhanced antibody binding to parasitized a-thalassemic cells [90, 91].

6. Erythrocnzymopathies

6.1 Glucose-6-phosphate dehydrogenase deficiency (G6PD)

Worldwide, one of the most frequent polymorphic disorders at the level of erythrocytes is the deficiency of glucose-6-phosphate dehydrogenase (G6PD), a condition that is triggered by the decrease in the activity of glucose-6-phosphate dehydrogenase [92]. This disorder linked to genetics is located in the terminal region of the long arm of chromosome X (Xq28) and characterized by establishing the condition of deficiency or normal in men; and in the case of women, it is established that they can be heterozygous, homozygous, or normal [92, 93]. The heterozygous women have a copy of the gene that synthesizes the normal G6PD and another copy that produces the variant of the enzyme.

The active enzyme consists of identical subunits that form dimers and tetramers, which contain a nicotinamide-adenine dinucleotide phosphate (NADP) binding site [94, 95]. NADP binds to the enzyme, as a structural component and as a substrate for the reaction. As shown in **Figure 4**, G6PD catalyzes the entry of glucose-6-phosphate (G6P) into the pentose phosphate pathway, specifically that of hexose monophosphate, a reaction that produces glucose-6 oxidation, phosphate to 6-phosphogluconolactone, reducing NADP to NADPH [96].

In erythrocytes, it is the only source of NADPH, being essential to protect cells against physiologically high levels of oxidative damage, enzymatic mechanisms associated with increases in reduced glutathione (GSH) [92]. Where glutaredoxin intervenes and by means of which GSH protects the sulfhydryl groups of the hemoglobin and the erythrocyte membrane, but in the presence of oxidizing agents, in the form of free radicals or peroxides, the level of GSH decreases, although it can be restored by the action of glutathione reductase which does have an adequate NADPH supplement [75].

Wide mechanisms have been described for the study of role of G6PD-deficiency as elements protective during infection with *P. falciparum*. The distribution in the world with respect to malaria is similar to the mutated alleles G6PD; these observations have evidenced that first studies evaluated the connection between G6PD deficiency and malaria, with contradictory results. However, the allelic heterogeneity of G6PD deficiency may be related with susceptibility of *P. falciparum* when infected erythrocytes are present under this condition. Thereby, studies established by Ruwende and col. have demonstrated that G6PD A- alleles are associated with a reduction in the risk of severe malaria caused by *P. falciparum*, protection that are confer principally in heterozygote individuals [97]. Likewise, experimental investigations have evidenced a diminution in the growth of parasitized-erythrocytes with G6PD A and A- in Mediterranean population when contrast with normal subject. Thus, this has indicated the incidence of mechanism of initial phagocytosis, where infected RBC of G6PD-deficicients is induced to phagocytosis by macrophages in anterior stages of the development of parasite, an aspect that is related with protective mechanism against malaria [98, 99]. Equally, a direct relationship of activation of process as phagocytosis in ring stages of parasite in erythrocytes infected with this condition has been considered [99]. This mechanism is associated with an increased binding of autologous IgG and complements C3 fragments when were compared with infected-RBC normal individuals [100]. Finally, have been associated a succession of phenomena's as the oxidation under increase of ROS into the erythrocytes and formation aggregated of band-3 protein [101].

6.2 Pyruvate kinase deficiency (PK)

Pyruvate kinase (PK) is an enzyme engaged in the conversion of phosphoenolpyruvate (PEP) to pyruvate. The catalysis of PK is an important element for formation of ATP in the glycolytic route [102]. PK plays a fundamental role in erythrocyte due to which cells depend on the production of ATP by glycolysis for the metabolic development and functionality of the cells [103]. The PK activity generally is increased in erythrocytes in the infection process. Likewise, have been associated to recognizing and the generation of the target of drug with *P. falciparum* infection [104]. PK deficiency is enzymatic alteration of the glycolytic route inducing non-spherocytic hemolytic anemia. The cause frequently linked is due to punctual mutations (1529A and 1456 T). PK deficiency presents worldwide distribution and is commonly prevalent in Caucasian populations [105].

It has been shown that PK deficiency is related to protection against infection in mice with *Plasmodium chabaudi* parasites, suggesting a similar effect of PK deficiency in humans. These effects have shown that PK-deficient human erythrocytes have induced diminution of malaria infection [106]. Other reports have indicated that possibly a protective effect against *P. falciparum* infection is generated, with alterations associated to replication on infected erythrocytes, where an invasive defect of erythrocytes in subjects bearing the homozygous mutation and to a preferential macrophage clearance of ring-infected erythrocytes is evidenced both in homozygous and heterozygous individuals [107].

Some phenomena have been associated with the deficiency of pyruvate kinase and infected erythrocytes, such as those established by the pleiotropic effect of the enzyme deficiency in the invasion of the parasite, which favors a substantial reduction of the growth of these and in the same way observes the activation of processes such as phagocytosis of infected erythrocytes in the ring stage that can provide protection against malaria, either by causing a reduction in the parasite burden or by reducing the number of erythrocytes infected with parasites in the trophozoites stages and schizonts that are available to join microvascular beds of vital organs [108].

These result in a reduced level of invasion of *P. falciparum* and erythrocytes of subjects with homozygous mutations. We also indicated that the possible biochemical differences in the intracellular medium, including the accumulation of glycolytic metabolic intermediates, did not cause a difference in the growth of parasites in erythrocytes between homozygotes and heterozygotes [109, 110]. To know even more the hypotheses of the reduction of the invasion observed in the erythrocytes of the subjects with homozygous mutations, it is also due to the capacity of the parasite, including the altered development of merozoites, the invasion of erythrocytes by merozoites was examined. It has been observed that the erythrocyte-tale merozoites had normal levels of invasion and replication in the erythrocytes of the control subjects [110].

We examined the phagocytic uptake of infected erythrocytes with *P. falciparum* (ring phase and mature phase) of case and control matter. Phagocytosis of infected erythrocytes in the ring stage of patients with homozygous mutations was higher than phagocytosis of uninfected erythrocytes. Also, an increased clearance has been observed by macrophages of erythrocytes infected in the ring stage of the parasite derivatives and heterozygotes for the PKLR mutation [108, 110].

Finally, it has led to establish that infected erythrocytes under this condition had a greater phagocytic phenomenon related to the development and deposition of hemichromes, IgG, and complement C3c [111, 112].

7. Conclusions

Malaria for years has been a study approach for scientists in the approach to the structural and functional study of the constituent proteins of the etiological agent, *Plasmodium falciparum*. A description of important proteins of the parasite has been established, as well as an approach of the main experimental studies that try to explain the molecular basis of each of the main erythrocyte polymorphisms shows a direct and significant resistance against the development of the parasite, and in this way, structural supports and detailed knowledge of some of these polymorphic modifications that show a complete field of study that will lead to the increasingly broad development of new tools for the compression and search for new pharmacological therapies are provided.

Acknowledgements

The author thanks University of Cartagena and Universitary Corporation Rafael Nuñez.

Conflict of interest

None.

Acronyms and abbreviations

AMA1	apical membrane antigen-1
CAT	catalase
CR1	complement receptor 1
C3c	complement component C3c
DBL	Duffy binding-like proteins
EDV	electron-dense vesicles
G6PD	glucose-6-phosphate dehydrogenase
GPI	glycosyl-phosphatidyl-inositol protein
GPX	glutathione peroxidase
GR	glutathione reductase
6PG	6-phosphogluconate dehydrogenase
GSH	glutathione reduced
GSSG	glutathione oxidized
HbAS	hemoglobin AS
IgG	immunoglobulin G
MC	Maurer's clefts
KHARP	Knobs-proteins rich in histidines
mi-RNA	micro-ribonucleic acid
MSP1	merozoite surface protein 1
NADP	nicotinamide-adenine dinucleotide phosphate
PV	parasitophorous vacuole
PVM	parasitophorous vacuole membrane
PfEMP1	*Plasmodium falciparum* erythrocyte membrane protein 1
PKLR	pyruvate kinase isozymes R/L
PK	pyruvate kinase
ROS	reactive oxygen species
RBP	reticulocyte binding proteins
SCT	sickle cell trait
TVN	tubulovesicular networks

Author details

Neyder Contreras-Puentes
University of Cartagena and Corporation Universitary Rafael Núñez, Cartagena, Colombia

*Address all correspondence to: neydercontreras11@gmail.com

References

[1] World Health Organization. World Malaria Report [Internet]. World Heal. Organ. 2016. pp. 1-186. Available from: http://apps.who.int/iris/bitstream/10665/252038/1/9789241511711-eng.pdf?ua=1

[2] De Mast Q, Brouwers J, Syafruddin D, Bousema T, Baidjoe AY, De Groot PG, et al. Is asymptomatic malaria really asymptomatic? Hematological, vascular and inflammatory effects of asymptomatic malaria parasitemia. The Journal of Infection. 2015;**71**(5):587-596. DOI: 10.1016/j.jinf.2015.08.005

[3] Bardach A, Ciapponi A, Rey-Ares L, Rojas JI, Mazzoni A, Glujovsky D, et al. Epidemiology of malaria in Latin America and the Caribbean from 1990 to 2009: Systematic review and meta-analysis. Value in Health Regional Issues. 2015;**8**:69-79. DOI: 10.1016/j.vhri.2015.05.002

[4] Goldberg DE, Cowman AF. Moving in and renovating: Exporting proteins from *Plasmodium* into host erythrocytes. Nature Reviews. Microbiology. 2010;**8**:617-621. DOI: 10.1038/nrmicro2420

[5] Tilley L, Dixon MWA, Kirk K. The *Plasmodium falciparum*-infected red blood cell. The International Journal of Biochemistry & Cell Biology. 2011;**43**(6):839-842. DOI: 10.1016/j.biocel.2011.03.012

[6] Maier AG, Cooke BM, Cowman AF, Tilley L. Malaria parasite proteins that remodel the host erythrocyte. Nature. 2009;**7**(5):341-54

[7] Mundwiler-pachlatko E, Beck H, Charles S, Alphonse L. Maurer's clefts, the enigma of *Plasmodium falciparum*. PNAS. 2013;**110**(50):19987-19994

[8] Spycher C, Rug M, Klonis N, Ferguson DJP, Cowman AF, Beck H-P, et al. Genesis of and trafficking to the Maurer's clefts of *Plasmodium falciparum*-infected erythrocytes. Molecular and Cellular Biology. 2006;**26**(11):4074-4085. DOI: 10.1128/MCB.00095-06

[9] Prajapati SK, Singh OP. Blood cells, molecules and diseases remodeling of human red cells infected with *Plasmodium falciparum* and the impact of PHIST proteins. Blood Cells, Molecules & Diseases. 2013;**51**(3):195-202. DOI: 10.1016/j.bcmd.2013.06.003

[10] Mohandas N, Gallagher PG. ASH 50th anniversary review red cell membrane: Past, present, and future. Blood. 2009;**112**(10):3939-3948

[11] Tomaiuolo G. Biomechanical properties of red blood cells in health and disease towards microfluidics. Biomicrofluidics. 2014;**8**(5):1-19. DOI: 10.1063/1.4895755

[12] Lu Y, Liu J. Erythrocyte membrane proteins and membrane skeleton. Frontiers of Biology in China. 2007;**2**(3):247-255

[13] Kakhniashvili D, Bulla L, Goodman S. The human erythrocyte proteome: Analysis by ion trap mass spectrometry. Molecular & Cellular Proteomics. 2004;**3**(5):501-509

[14] Wright GJ, Rayner JC. *Plasmodium falciparum* erythrocyte invasion: Combining function with immune evasion. PLoS Pathogens. 2014;**10**(3):1-7

[15] Mazumdar S, Mukherjee P, Yazdani SS, Jain SK, Mohmmed A, Chauhan VS. *Plasmodium falciparum* merozoite surface protein 1 (MSP-1)-MSP-3 chimeric protein: Immunogenicity determined with human-compatible adjuvants and induction of protective immune response. Infection and Immunity. 2010;**78**(2):872-883

[16] Das S, Hertrich N, Perrin AJ, Withers-Martinez C, Collins CR, Jones ML, et al. Processing of *Plasmodium falciparum* Merozoite surface protein MSP1 activates a Spectrin-binding function enabling parasite egress from RBCs. Cell Host & Microbe. 2015;**18**(4):433-444. DOI: 10.1016/j.chom.2015.09.007

[17] Beeson JG, Drew DR, Boyle MJ, Feng G, Fowkes FJI, Richards JS. Merozoite surface proteins in red blood cell invasion, immunity and vaccines against malaria. FEMS Microbiology Reviews. 2016;**40**(3):343-372

[18] Cowman AF, Crabb BS. Invasion of red blood cells by malaria parasites. Cell. 2006;**124**(4):755-766

[19] Kinoshita T. Glycosylphosphatidylinositol (GPI) anchors: Biochemistry and cell biology: Introduction to a thematic review series. Journal of Lipid Research. 2016;**57**(1):4-5. DOI: 10.1194/jlr.E065417

[20] Srinivasan P, Beatty WL, Diouf A, Herrera R, Ambroggio X, Moch JK, et al. Binding of Plasmodium merozoite proteins RON2 and AMA1 triggers commitment to invasion. Proceedings of the National Academy of Sciences. 2011;**108**(32):13275-13280. DOI: 10.1073/pnas.1110303108

[21] Yang ASP, Lopaticki S, O'Neill MT, Erickson SM, Douglas DN, Kneteman NM, et al. AMA1 and MAEBL are important for *Plasmodium falciparum* sporozoite infection of the liver. Cellular Microbiology. 2017;**19**(9):e12745

[22] Tolia NH, Enemark EJ, Sim BKL, Joshua-tor L. Structural basis for the EBA-175 erythrocyte invasion pathway of the malaria parasite *Plasmodium falciparum*. Cell. 2005;**122**:183-193

[23] Lopaticki S, Maier AG, Thompson J, Wilson DW, Tham WH, Triglia T, et al. Reticulocyte and erythrocyte binding-like proteins function cooperatively in invasion of human erythrocytes by malaria parasites. Infection and Immunity. 2011;**79**(3):1107-1117

[24] Li X, Marinkovic M, Russo C, McKnight CJ, Coetzer TL, Chishti AH. Identification of a specific region of *Plasmodium falciparum* EBL-1 that binds to host receptor glycophorin B and inhibits merozoite invasion in human red blood cells. Molecular and Biochemical Parasitology. 2012;**183**(1):23-31

[25] Richard D, Macraild CA, Riglar DT, Chan J, Foley M, Baum J, et al. Interaction between *Plasmodium falciparum* apical membrane antigen 1 and the Rhoptry neck protein complex defines a key step in the erythrocyte invasion process of malaria parasites. The Journal of Biological Chemistry. 2010;**285**(19):14815-14822

[26] Méndez D. Proteómica Redox De Membrana De Eritrocito Humano En Malaria Y Polimorfismos De Grupos Sanguíneos Y G6PD. 2011

[27] Mbengue A, Yam XY, Braun-Breton C. Human erythrocyte remodelling during *Plasmodium falciparum* malaria parasite growth and egress. British Journal of Haematology. 2012;**157**(2):171-179

[28] Morse D, Webster W, Kalanon M, Langsley G, McFadden GI. *Plasmodium falciparum* Rab1A localizes to rhoptries in schizonts. PLoS One. 2016;**11**(6):1-13

[29] Lang PA, Kasinathan RS, Brand VB, Lang C, Koka S, Shumilina E, et al. Accelerated clearance of Plasmodium-infected erythrocytes in sickle cell trait and Annexin-A7 deficiency. Cellular Physiology and Biochemistry. 2009;**24**:415-428

[30] Zuccala ES, Baum J. Cytoskeletal and membrane remodelling during

malaria parasite invasion of the human erythrocyte. British Journal of Haematology. 2011;**154**(July):680-689

[31] Martinez SL, Clavijo CA, Winograd E. Identification of peripheral membrane proteins associated with the tubo-vesicular network of *Plasmodium falciparum* infected erythrocytes. Molecular and Biochemical Parasitology. 1998;**91**(2):273-280

[32] Cooke BM, Mohandas N, Coppel RL. The malaria-infected red blood cell: Structural and functional changes. Advances in Parasitology. 2001;**50**:1-86

[33] Deponte M, Hoppe HC, Lee MCS, Maier AG, Richard D, Rug M, et al. Molecular & biochemical parasitology wherever I may roam: Protein and membrane trafficking in *P. falciparum*-infected red blood cells. Molecular and Biochemical Parasitology. 2012;**186**:95-116. DOI: 10.1016/j.molbiopara.2012.09.007

[34] Mcmillan PJ, Millet C, Batinovic S, Maiorca M, Kenny S, Muhle RA, et al. Spatial and temporal mapping of the PfEMP1 export in pathway *Plasmodium falciparum*. NIH Public Access. 2014;**15**(8):1401-1418

[35] Rug M, Prescott SW, Fernandez KM, Cooke BM, Cowman AF. The role of KAHRP domains in knob formation and cytoadherence of *P. falciparum*-infected human erythrocytes. Blood. 2006;**108**(1):370-378

[36] Chen Q, Schlichtherle M, Wahlgren M. Molecular aspects of severe malaria. Clinical Microbiology Reviews. 2000;**13**(3):439-450

[37] Goyal M, Alam A, Bandyopadhyay U. Redox regulation in malaria: Current concepts and Pharmacotherapeutic implications. Current Medicinal Chemistry. 2012;**19**:1475-1503

[38] Yam XY, Mbengue A, Braun-breton C. Human erythrocyte remodelling by *Plasmodium falciparum*. In: Malaria Parasites. Intechopen. 2012. pp. 107-135

[39] Smith JD, Rowe JA, Higgins MK, Lavstsen T. Microreview Malaria's deadly grip: Cytoadhesion of *Plasmodium falciparum*-infected erythrocytes. Cellular microbiology. 2013;**15**(12):1976-1983

[40] Waller KL, Nunomura W, An X, Cooke BM, Mohandas N, Coppel RL. Brief report Mature parasite-infected erythrocyte surface antigen (MESA) of *Plasmodium falciparum* binds to the 30-kDa domain of protein 4.1 in malaria-infected red blood cells. Blood. 2003;**102**(5):1911-1914

[41] Pei X, Guo X, Coppel R, Mohandas N, An X. *Plasmodium falciparum* erythrocyte membrane protein 3 (PfEMP3) destabilizes erythrocyte membrane skeleton. The Journal of Biological Chemistry. 2007;**282**(37):26754-26758

[42] Enderle T, Ha T, Ogletree DF, Chemla DS, Magowan C, Weiss S. Membrane specific mapping and colocalization of malarial and host skeletal proteins in the *Plasmodium falciparum* infected erythrocyte by dual-color near-field scanning optical microscopy. Proceedings of the National Academy of Sciences of the United States of America. 1997;**94**(2):520-525

[43] Cooke BM, Mohandas N, Coppel RL. Malaria and the red blood cell membrane. Seminars in Hematology. 2004;**41**(2):173-188

[44] Spielmann T, Gilberger T. Critical steps in protein export of *Plasmodium falciparum* blood stages. Trends in Parasitology. 2015;**31**(10):514-525. DOI: 10.1016/j.pt.2015.06.010

[45] Magowan C, Nunomura W, Waller KL, Yeung J, Liang J, Van Dort H, et al.

Plasmodium falciparum histidine-rich protein 1 associates with the band 3 binding domain of ankyrin in the infected red cell membrane. Biochmica Biophys Acta. 2000;**1502**(3):461-470

[46] Jobe SM, Wilson KM, Leo L, Raimondi A, Molkentin JD, Steven R, et al. Critical role for the mitochondrial permeability transition pore and cyclophilin D in platelet activation and thrombosis. Blood. 2014;**111**(3):1257-1265

[47] Zhang M, Faou P, Maier AG, Rug M. *Plasmodium falciparum* exported protein PFE60 influences Maurer's clefts architecture and virulence complex composition. International Journal for Parasitology. 2017;**48**(1):83-95. DOI: 10.1016/j.ijpara.2017.09.003

[48] Nolte D, Hundt E, Langsley G, Knapp B. A *Plasmodium falciparum* blood stage antigen highly homologous to the glycophorin binding protein GBP. Molecular and Biochemical Parasitology. 1991;**49**(2):253-264

[49] Knuepfer E, Rug M, Klonis N, Tilley L, Cowman AF. Trafficking determinants for PfEMP3 export and assembly under the *Plasmodium falciparum*-infected red blood cell membrane. Molecular Microbiology. 2005;**58**(4):1039-1053

[50] Pasternak ND, Dzikowski R. PfEMP1: An antigen that plays a key role in the pathogenicity and immune evasion of the malaria parasite *Plasmodium falciparum*. The International Journal of Biochemistry & Cell Biology. 2009;**41**(7): 1463-1466. Available from: http://linkinghub.elsevier.com/retrieve/pii/S1357272508005098

[51] Niang M, Yam XY, Preiser PR. The *Plasmodium falciparum* STEVOR multigene family mediates antigenic variation of the infected erythrocyte. PLoS Pathogens. 2009;**5**(2):e1000307

[52] Deponte M, Hoppe HC, Lee MCS, Maier AG, Richard D, Rug M, et al. Molecular & biochemical parasitology wherever I may roam: Protein and membrane trafficking in *P. falciparum*-infected red blood cells. Molecular and Biochemical Parasitology. 2012;**186**(2):95-116. DOI: 10.1016/j.molbiopara.2012.09.007

[53] Spycher C, Klonis N, Spielmann T, Kump E, Steiger S, Tilley L, et al. MAHRP-1, a novel *Plasmodium falciparum* histidine-rich protein, binds ferriprotoporphyrin IX and localizes to the Maurer's clefts. The Journal of Biological Chemistry. 2003;**278**(37):35373-35383

[54] Mchugh E, Batinovic S, Hanssen E, Mcmillan PJ, Kenny S, Griffin MDW, et al. A repeat sequence domain of the ring-exported protein-1 of *Plasmodium falciparum* controls export machinery architecture and virulence protein trafficking. Molecular Microbiology. 2015;**98**(6):1101-1114

[55] Cserti CM, Dzik WH. The ABO blood group system and Plasmodium falciparum malaria. Blood. 2007;**110**(7):2250-2258. DOI: 10.1182/blood-2007-03-077602

[56] Sabbatani S, Manfredi R, Fiorino S. Malaria infection and the anthropological evolution. Saúde e Soc. 2010;**19**(1):64-83. Available from: http://www.scielo.br/scielo.php?script=sci_arttext&pid=S0104-12902010000100006&lng=en&tlng=en

[57] Bauduer F. Red cell polymorphisms and malaria: An evolutionary approach. Bulletins et mémoires de la Société d'Anthropologie de Paris. 2013;**25**(1-2):55-64

[58] Cyrklaff M, Sanchez CP, Frischknecht F, Lanzer M. Host actin remodeling and protection from malaria by hemoglobinopathies. Trends in

Parasitology. 2012;**28**(11):479-485. DOI: 10.1016/j.pt.2012.08.003

[59] López C, Saravia C, Gomez A, Hoebeke J, Patarroyo MA. Mechanisms of genetically-based resistance to malaria. Gene. 2010;**467**(1-2):1-12. Available from: http://linkinghub.elsevier.com/retrieve/pii/S0378111910002933

[60] Modell B, Darlison M. Global epidemiology of haemoglobin disorders and derived service indicators. Bulletin of the World Health Organization. 2008;**86**(6):480-487

[61] Weatherall DJ, Clegg JB. Inherited haemoglobin disorders: An increasing global health problem. Bulletin of the World Health Organization. 2001;**79**(8):704-712. Available from: /pmc/articles/PMC2566499/?report=abstract

[62] Domínguez Y, Zurita C, Calvopiña D, Villacís J, Mora M. Prevalence of common hemoglobin variants in an afro-descendent Ecuadorian population. BMC Research Notes. 2013;**6**(1):132. Available from: http://www.biomedcentral.com/1756-0500/6/132

[63] Yusuf HR, Lloyd-Puryear MA, Grant AM, Parker CS, Creary MS, Atrash HK. Sickle cell disease. American Journal of Preventive Medicine. 2011;**41**(6):S376-S383. Available from: http://linkinghub.elsevier.com/retrieve/pii/S0749379711006209

[64] Alvear CC, Barboza M, Viola M, Moneriz C, Araque LM. Pilot study of hemoglobinopathies in newborns of the Rafael Calvo maternity clinic of Cartagena, Colombia. Estud Pilot hemoglobinopatías en recién nacidos la Clínica Matern Rafael Calvo Cart Colomb. 2012;**43**(3):196-199. Available from: http://search.ebscohost.com/login.aspx?direct=true&db=a9h&AN=82559076&lang=es&site=ehost-live

[65] de Mendonça VRR, Goncalves MS, Barral-Netto M. The host genetic diversity in malaria infection. Journal of Tropical Medicine. 2012;**2012**:1-17. Available from: http://www.hindawi.com/journals/jtm/2012/940616/

[66] Hedrick PW. Population genetics of malaria resistance in humans. Heredity (Edinb). 2011;**107**:283-304. DOI: 10.1038/hdy.2011.16

[67] Voskou S, Aslan M, Fanis P, Phylactides M, Kleanthous M. Oxidative stress in β-thalassaemia and sickle cell disease. Redox Biology. 2015;**6**:226-239. DOI: 10.1016/j.redox.2015.07.018

[68] Rees DC, Williams TN, Gladwin MT. Sickle-cell disease. Lancet. 2010;**376**(9757):2018-2031. DOI: 10.1016/S0140-6736(10)61029-X

[69] Ware KM, Feinstein DL, Rubinstein I, Battula P, Otero J, Hebert L, et al. The severity of intracranial hemorrhages measured by free hemoglobin in the brain depends on the anticoagulant class: Experimental data. Stroke Research and Treatment. 2017;**2017**:1-4

[70] Ferreira A, Balla J, Jeney V, Balla G, Soares MP. A central role for free heme in the pathogenesis of severe malaria: The missing link? Journal of Molecular Medicine. 2008;**86**(10):1097-1111

[71] Kilian N, Srismith S, Dittmer M, Ouermi D, Bisseye C, Simpore J, et al. Hemoglobin S and C affect protein export in *Plasmodium falciparum* -infected erythrocytes. Biology Open. 2015:400-410

[72] Alayash AI. Hemoglobin-based blood substitutes and the treatment of sickle cell disease: More harm than help? Biomolecules. 2017;**7**(1):1-13

[73] Jana S, Meng F, Hirsch RE, Friedman JM, Alayash AI. Oxidized mutant human hemoglobins S and E induce oxidative stress and bioenergetic

dysfunction in human pulmonary endothelial cells. Frontiers in Physiology. 2017;**8**(Dec):1-14

[74] Pasvol G, Weatherall D, Wilson R. Cellular mechanism for the protective effect of haemoglobin S against *P. falciparum* malaria. Nature. 1978;**274**(5672):701-703

[75] Pasvol G, Weatherall DJ. The red cell and the malarial parasite. British Journal of Haematology. 1980;**46**(2):165-170

[76] Archer NM, Petersen N, Clark MA, Buckee CO, Childs LM, Duraisingh MT. Resistance to *Plasmodium falciparum* in sickle cell trait erythrocytes is driven by oxygen-dependent growth inhibition. Proceedings of the National Academy of Sciences. 2018:201804388. DOI: 10.1073/pnas.1804388115

[77] Aneni EC, Hamer DH, Gill CJ. Systematic review of current and emerging strategies for reducing morbidity from malaria in sickle cell disease. Tropical Medicine & International Health. 2013;**18**(3): 313-327. Available from: http://www.ncbi.nlm.nih.gov/pubmed/23320577

[78] Williams TN. Human red blood cell polymorphisms and malaria. Current Opinion in Microbiology. 2006;**9**:388-394

[79] Becker K, Tilley L, Vennerstrom JL, Roberts D, Rogerson S, Ginsburg H. Oxidative stress in malaria parasite-infected erythrocytes: Host-parasite interactions. International Journal for Parasitology. 2004;**34**:163-189. Available from: http://linkinghub.elsevier.com/retrieve/pii/S002075190300314X

[80] Ayi K, Turrini F, Piga A, Arese P. Enhanced phagocytosis of ring-parasitized mutant erythrocytes: A common mechanism that may explain protection against falciparum malaria in sickle trait and beta-thalassemia trait. Blood. 2004;**104**(10):3364-3371. Available from: http://www.ncbi.nlm.nih.gov/pubmed/15280204

[81] Bunn HF. The triumph of good over evil: Protection by the sickle gene against malaria. Blood. 2013;**121**(1):20-25

[82] Luzzi GA, Merry AH, Newbold CI, Marsh KI, Pasvol G. Protection by a-thalassaemia against *Plasmodium falciparum* malaria: Modified surface antigen expression rather than impaired growth or cytoadherence. Immunology Letters. 1991;**30**:233-240

[83] Mockenhaupt FP, Ehrhardt S, Gellert S, Otchwemah RN, Dietz E, Anemana SD, et al. Brief report α+−thalassemia protects African children from severe malaria. Blood. 2004;**104**(7):2003-2007

[84] Krause MA, Diakite SAS, Lopera-mesa TM, Amaratunga C, Arie T, Traore K, et al. A -thalassemia impairs the Cytoadherence of *Plasmodium falciparum*-infected erythrocytes methods. PLoS One. 2012;**7**(5):1-7

[85] Premawardhena A, Arambepola M, Samaranayake R, Allen SJ, Peto TEA, Fisher CA, et al. Interaction of malaria with a common form of severe thalassemia in an Asian population. PNAS. 2009;**106**(4):18716-18721

[86] Mockenhaupt FP, Bienzle U, Falusi AG, Ademowo OG, Olumese PE, Meyer CG. *Plasmodium falciparum* infection: Influence on hemoglobin levels in a -thalassemia and Microcytosis. The Journal of Infectious Diseases. 1999;**180**(September):925-928

[87] Ayi K, Turrini F, Piga A, Arese P. Enhanced phagocytosis of ring-parasitized mutant erythrocytes: A common mechanism that may explain protection against falciparum malaria in sickle trait and beta-thalassemia trait. Blood. 2004;**104**(10):3364-3372

[88] Roberts DJ, Williams TN, Roberts DJ, Williams TN. Haemoglobinopathies and resistance to malaria. Redox Report. 2013;**8**(5):2003

[89] Cockburn IA, Mackinnon MJ, Donnell AO, Allen SJ, Moulds JM, Baisor M, et al. A human complement receptor 1 polymorphism that reduces *Plasmodium falciparum* rosetting confers protection against severe malaria. PNAS. 2003;**101**(1):272-277

[90] Para S, Mungkalasut P, Chanda M, Nuchprayoon I, Krudsood S, Cheepsunthorn CL. An observational study of the effect of hemoglobinopathy, alpha thalassemia and hemoglobin E on P. Vivax Parasitemia. Mediterranean Journal of Hematology and Infectious Diseases. 2018;**10**(1):e2018015

[91] Williams TN, Wambua S, Uyoga S, Macharia A, Mwacharo JK, Newton CRJC. Brief report both heterozygous and homozygousm α+thalassemias protect against severe and fatal *Plasmodium falciparum* malaria on the coast of Kenya. Blood. 2005;**106**(1):368-372

[92] Cappellini MD, Fiorelli G. Glucose-6-phosphate dehydrogenase deficiency. Lancet. 2008;**371**(9606):64-74

[93] Luzzatto L. Glucose 6-phosphate dehydrogenase deficiency: From genotype to phenotype. Haematologica. 2006;**91**(10):1303-1306

[94] Fonseca D, Mateus H, Silva C, Contreras N, Restrepo C. Deficiencia de glucosa 6-fosfato deshidrogenasa: Aspectos generales de la eritroenzimopatía más frecuente en el mundo. Acta Médica Colombiana. 2005;**30**(2):59-64

[95] Stanton RC. Glucose-6-phosphate dehydrogenase, NADPH, and cell survival. IUBMB Life. 2012;**64**(5): 362-369. DOI: 10.1002/iub.1017

[96] Bonilla J, Sánchez M, Chuaire L. Glucosa-6-fosfato deshidrogenasa (G6PD). Respuesta de los hematíes y otras células humanas a la disminución en su actividad. Colombia Médica. 2007;**38**:68-75. Available from: http://scholar.google.com/scholar?hl=en&btnG=Search&q=intitle:Glucosa-6-fosfato+deshidrogenasa+(+G6PD+).+Respuesta+de+los+hematíes+y+otras+células+humanas+a+la+disminución+en+su+actividad#0

[97] Ruwende C, Hill A. Glucose-6-phosphate dehydrogenase deficiency and malaria. Journal of Molecular Medicine. 1998;**76**(8):581-588. Available from: http://www.ncbi.nlm.nih.gov/pubmed/9694435

[98] Allahverdiyev AM, Bagirova M, Elcicek S. Glucose-6-Phosphate Dehydrogenase Deficiency and Malaria: A Method to Detect Primaquine-Induced Hemolysis in Vitro. Intechopen; 2012

[99] Ginsburg H, Atamna H, Shalmiev G, Kanaani J, Krugliak M. Resistance of glucose-6-phosphate dehydrogenase deficiency to malaria: Effects of fava bean hydroxypyrimidine glucosides on *Plasmodium falciparum* growth in culture and on the phagocytosis of infected cells. Parasitology. 1996;(113(Pt.1)):7-18

[100] Hwang S, Mruk K, Rahighi S, Raub AG, Chen C, Dorn LE, et al. Correcting glucose-6-phosphate dehydrogenase deficiency with a small-molecule activator. Nature Communications. 2018;**9**(1):1-12

[101] Luzzatto L, Arese P. Favism and glucose-6-phosphate dehydrogenase deficiency. The New England Journal of Medicine. 2018;**378**(1):60-71. DOI: 10.1056/NEJMra1708111

[102] Grace RF, Zanella A, Neufeld EJ, Morton DH, Eber S, Yaish H, et al. Erythrocyte pyruvate kinase deficiency:

2015 status report. American Journal of Hematology. 2015;**90**(9):825-830

[103] Zanella A, Fermo E, Bianchi P, Valentini G. Red cell pyruvate kinase deficiency: Molecular and clinical aspects. British Journal of Haematology. 2005;**130**:11-25

[104] Abdrhamn B, Gibreel M. Human genetic factors associated with protection against malaria. Iraqi Journal of Hematology. 2018;7:97-98

[105] Machado P, Manco L, Gomes C, Mendes C, Fernandes N, Salomé G, et al. Pyruvate kinase deficiency in sub-Saharan Africa: Identification of a highly frequent missense mutation (G829A; Glu277Lys) and association with malaria. PLoS One. 2012:7(10)

[106] Min-oo G, Fortin A, Tam M, Nantel A, Stevenson MM, Gros P. Pyruvate kinase deficiency in mice protects against malaria. Nature Genetics. 2003;**35**(4):357-362

[107] Ayi K, Liles WC, Gros P, Kain KC. Adenosine triphosphate depletion of erythrocytes simulates the phenotype associated with pyruvate kinase deficiency and confers protection against *Plasmodium falciparum* In vitro. The Journal of Infectious Diseases. 2009;**200**:1289-1299

[108] van Bruggen RCG, Iliescu A, Cheepsunthorn CL, Mungkalasut P, Trape J-F, Modiano D, et al. Modulation of malaria phenotypes by pyruvate kinase (PKLR) variants in a Thai. Population. 2015:1-18

[109] Min-Oo G, Fortin A, Tam M-F, Gros P, Stevenson M. Phenotypic expression of pyruvate kinase deficiency and protection against malaria in a mouse model. Genes and Immunity. 2004;**5**(3):168-175

[110] Crockett M, Kirby-allen M, Quirt I, Gros P, Ph D, Kain KC. Pyruvate kinase deficiency and malaria. The New England Journal of Medicine. 2008;**358**(17):1805-1810

[111] Petz LD, Yam P, Wilkinson L, Garratty G, Lubin B, Mentzer W. Increased IgG molecules bound to the surface of red blood cells of patients with sickle cell anemia. Blood. 1984;**64**(1):301-304

[112] Skardoutsou A, Voudris KA, Mastroyianni S, Vagiakou E, Magoufis G, Koukoutsakis P. Moya Moya syndrome in a child with pyruvate kinase deficiency and combined prothrombotic factors. Journal of Child Neurology. 2007;**22**(4):474-478

Chapter 4

Pharmacokinetic and Pharmacodynamic Profiles of Rapid- and Slow-Acting Antimalarial Drugs

Qigui Li and Brandon Pybus

Abstract

Artemisinin and its derivatives are highly effective antimalarial drugs. These compounds combine potent and rapid antimalarial activity with a wide therapeutic index. An initiation of artemisinin resistance, described by a delayed parasite clearance time, is unlikely to cause high-level resistance. Artemisinins as a class demonstrate poor efficacy as monotherapy. This shortcoming can be overcome using oral artemisinin-based combination therapies (ACT) and intravenous-artesunate (IV-AS) in combination with slow-acting partner drugs. Pharmacokinetic and pharmacodynamic (PK/PD) evaluation demonstrates that the rapid efficacy of artemisinins is largely due to drug peak concentrations. Critical evaluation also demonstrates that AS is superior in PK/PD either following oral or intravenous administration when compared to the other rapid-acting artemisinins. This rapid efficacy and decreased mortality demonstrates that currently available artemisinins have a great advantage when combined with slow-acting antimalarial drugs for uncomplicated malaria or in sequential therapy with AS injection initially for severe and complicated malaria. Compared to other ACTs, dihydroartemisinin-piperaquine (DP) demonstrates a superior in PK/PD profile, most likely due to the long half-life of piperaquine. These findings will help us better understand the PK/PD profiles of rapid-acting (artemisinins) and slow-acting (piperaquine) drugs, and suggest how to best use ACTs in the future.

Keywords: artemisinin, artesunate, piperaquine, pharmacokinetics, pharmacodynamics

1. Introduction

The artemisinin group of antimalarials is considered to be highly and rapidly effective compared with other traditional malaria drugs. Resistance to artemisinins emerged in 2008 in parts of Southeast Asia and continues to spread [1]. Although there is more evidence to confirm drug resistance [2, 3], artemisinin and its derivatives are still widely used in current malaria therapy [2, 4]. Clinical artemisinin resistance is demonstrated as a delayed clearance phenotype; that is, infection finally resolves with treatment with artemisinin-based combination therapies (ACTs), but the time required for parasite clearance substantially increases [5].

High rates of recrudescence with daily monotherapy of artemisinins for 3–5 days are observed in humans. However, this shortfall is being overcome using oral ACTs and injectable artesunate (IV-AS) in combination with slow-acting antimalarial drugs. The rapid parasite killing of artemisinins in the treatment of early uncomplicated malaria with ACTs may prevent its progression to more severe disease with subsequent reduction in severe cases and associated mortality [6]. ACTs are currently the preferred treatment for malaria due to their enhanced efficacy and the potential to lower the emergence and spread of resistance [7].

The WHO has endorsed ACTs as the "policy standard" for all malaria infections in areas where *P. falciparum* is the predominant infecting species. Four ACTs recommended by a WHO Expert Consultative Group in 2001 are artemether (AM)-lumefantrine (Coartem), AS-mefloquine (Artequin), AS-amodiaquine, and AS-sulfadoxine/pyrimethamine [8]. Monotherapy with the artemisinins was significantly decreased after 2001 to prevent the emergence of resistance. However, IV-AS, as a monotherapy, is still in first line of treatment for both adults and children in Asian countries [9] for complicated and severe malaria, as well as some areas in Africa [10].

Recent trials have used IV-AS with its more favorable pharmacokinetic profile [11, 12]. The SEAQUAMAT trial, a large multicenter randomized trial carried out in Bangladesh, Thailand, Myanmar, Indonesia, India, and Vietnam, showed a 34.7% reduction in mortality from all causes associated with IV-AS as compared to intravenous quinine [13]. This remains the largest trial performed for severe malaria and was the first to conclusively demonstrate a benefit over standard quinine therapy. There is strong evidence that IV-AS will reduce the risk of death by one-third when compared to quinine therapy in cases of severe malaria. Consequently, IV-AS was immediately recommended for patients with severe malaria by The European Network on Imported Infections Disease Surveillance (TropNetEurop) after these trials [14].

The most recent development in antimalarial therapy is the use of artemisinin derivatives, especially IV-AS, which will potentially revolutionize the management of severe and complicated [15]. Therefore, there is a strong case for continued need for AS as a monotherapy, if only for this niche indication [16]. However, there is currently no useable formulation available that is produced under good manufacturing practice (GMP) conditions. The Walter Reed Army Institute of Research (WRAIR) continues to develop a novel cGMP injection of AS since 2004, which is in the process of US FDA approval [17, 18].

2. PK/PD evaluation of the artemisinins in patients

Pharmacokinetics (PK), in general, comprises three distinct phases (absorption, distribution, and elimination) of artemisinin drugs in blood after oral, intravenous, or intramuscular administration. Following single oral administration, AS and dihydroartemisinin (DHA) have short mean residence times (MRT) of 2.0 and 2.7 h, respectively, and artemisinin (QHS) has a longer MRT of 7.4 h. Following intramuscular injections, arteether (AE) and AM both display very long MRTs at 13.9 and 42.9 h respectively. However, IV-AS displays the shortest MRT (0.90 h) after intravenous injection (**Table 1**). It is obvious that the different artemisinins and the method of their delivery result in significant differences in PK characteristics in humans. After multiple administrations, four drug concentrations of QHS, DHA, AS, and AM have been reported to decline daily due to autoinduction metabolism [19–23] that may result in the high rates of recrudescence with the monotherapy at a multiple dosing.

Pharmacodynamics (PD) has similarities to PK profiles but instead measures parameters of efficacy. For any antimalarial, the mean parasitemia-time curve

PK/PD parameters	AS [25–27]	AS [22, 28, 29]	DHA [30–32]	QHS [33, 34]	AM [35–37]	AE [37–39]
Route of administration	Intravenous	Oral	Oral	Oral	Intramuscular	Intramuscular
First loading dosage	120 mg	100 mg	200 mg	500 mg	3.2 mg/kg	4.8 mg/kg
Maintaining dosage	Oral 100 mg at 8 h	50 mg b.i.d. × 4	100 mg × 4	250 × 2 × 5	1.6 mg/kg × 4	1.6 mg/kg × 5
Total dose	220 mg and mefloquine**	500 mg	600 mg	3000 mg	9.6 mg/kg	12.8 mg/kg
PK parameters (day 1)						
C_{max} (ng/ml)	2646 (DHA); 11,343(AS)	1052 (DHA); 198 (AS)	437.5	588.0	74.9	110.1
T_{max} (h)	0.13	0.75	1.4	2.4	6.0	8.2
T_{lag} (h)			0.2	0.45		
$AUC_{0–24\,h}$ (ng h/ml)	2378 (DHA); 1146 (AS)	1334 (DHA); 210 (AS)	1329	2601	1230	4702
$t_{1/2}$ (absorption, h)	—	0.36 (DHA)	0.67	1.21	1.88	3.2
$t_{1/2}$ (elimination, h)	0.67 (DHA); 0.05 (AS)	0.70 (DHA)	0.85	2.3	7.83	22.7
MRT (h)	0.90 (DHA)	1.95 (DHA)	2.71	7.41	13.94	42.9
PD parameters (day 1)*						
Time of lag phase (h)	1.92	2.81	4.03	5.76	7.26	8.89
AUIC (% h/µl)	397.3	921.2	1167.9	1464.4	1613.4	2463.5
PC_{50} (h)	3.18	8.48	10.05	13.95	15.63	19.68
E_{max} (%) or MPC	0.0011	0.0016	0.2132	0.0100	0.0030	0.5504
Curative rate (%)	100**	81.3	76.0	74.3	86.7	48.0

The data was fitted with WinNonlin (V5.0) by author.

***Oral 750 mg mefloquine at 24 h after IV injection. PK = pharmacokinetics; PD = pharmacodynamics; MRT = mean residence time; PC_{50} = mean time for parasitemia to fall by half; AUIC = area under inhibitory curve; QHS = artemisinin; DHA = dihydroartemisinin; AM = artemether; AE = arteether; AS = artesunic acid; MPC = minimum parasiticidal concentration; IM = intramuscular.*

Table 1.
Pharmacokinetics/pharmacodynamics (PK/PD) parameters of IV-AS (IV 120 mg and oral 100 mg at 8 h, then oral 750 mg mefloquine at 24 h), AS (oral, 100 mg and then 50 mg b.i.d × 4), DHA (oral, 200 mg and then 100 mg × 4), QHS (oral, 500 mg and 250 b.i.d × 4 and then 500 mg on D6), AM (IM, 3.2 mg/kg and 1.6 mg × 4), and AE (IM, 4.8 mg/kg at 0 h and 1.6 mg/kg at 6 h and then day 2–5 daily) in human treatment with uncomplicated and severe/complicated malaria on day 1.*

following administration presents as a lag phase. This lag phase is then followed by a sharp drop in parasite burden (representing the clearance phase), which is then followed by a slow decrease to very low parasitemia levels. Subsequent phases of this process are usually under the limits of microscopic detection of both the dormant and terminal phases (**Figure 1**, top). The artemisinins affect this profile in multiple ways. First, they prevent the continuation of merogony at later stages of parasite development as compared to quinine or mefloquine. This stops the occasional alarming sharp rise in parasitemia immediately following treatment described earlier (lag phase).

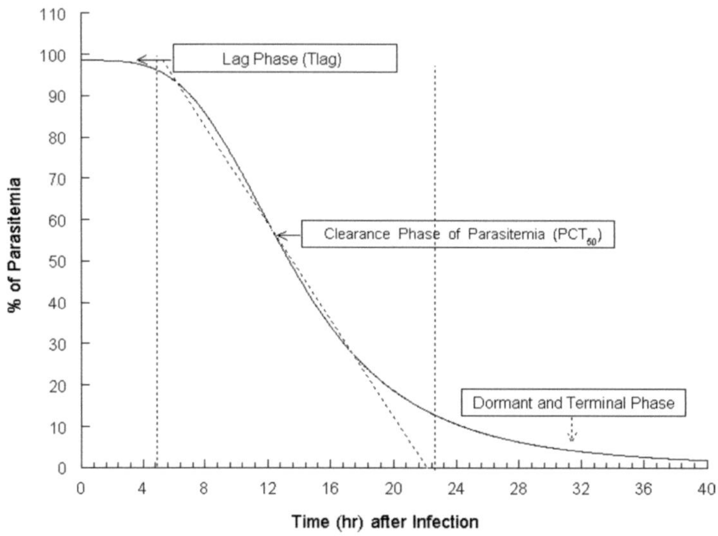

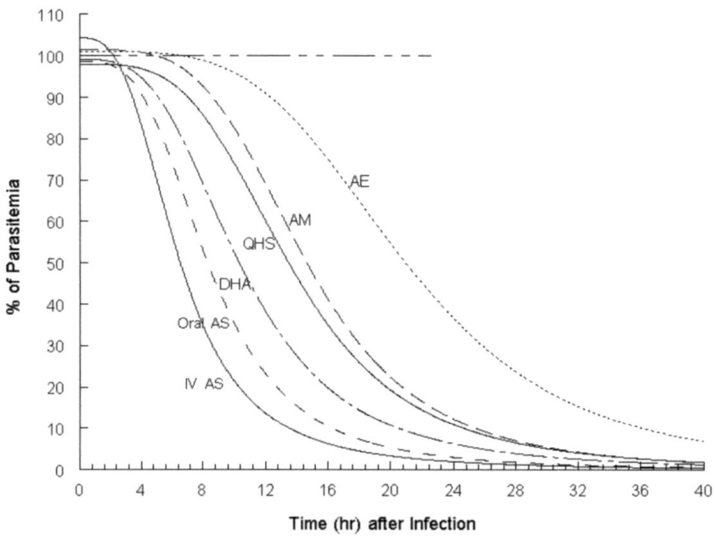

Figure 1.
*Standard parasite clearance curve in different stages (lag phase, clearance phase, dormant and terminal phase) and synchronicity of parasite development under antiparasitic drug received at 0 h (top chart). The mean parasite clearance curves (bottom chart) of AS (solid line) at single intravenous 120 mg and oral 100 mg at 8 h, then oral 750 mg mefloquine at 24 h [26, 27]; oral AS (dashed line) at 100 mg first day and 50 mg b.i.d 2–5 days orally [22, 28, 29]; oral DHA (dot and dashed line) at 200 mg first day and 100 mg 2–5 days orally [30, 31]; oral QHS (solid line) at 500 mg first day, 250 mg b.i.d 2–5 and 500 mg last day orally [19–21, 29]; intramuscular AM (dashed line) at 3.2 mg/kg first day and 1.6 mg/kg 2–5 days intramuscularly [35, 36]; and intramuscular AE (dot line) of 4.8 mg/kg at 0 h and 1.6 mg/kg at 6 and then 2–5 days intramuscularly [38, 39], in malaria patients (bottom chart) (**Table 1**). The parasitemia at 0 h was set as 100% of parasitemia.*

Second, the drop in parasite load is accelerated. This is explained by enhanced clearance of erythrocytes infected with ring forms (clearance phase) [24]. Rapid termination, surviving and stage unaffected parasites display very low levels of dormancy [25], which is the basis of the recrudescence (dormant and terminal phase). Different artemisinins with varied methods of delivery show different parasitemia-time profiles (**Figure 1**, bottom). Although the PK/PD publication record is very limited, the possible PK and PD evaluations for individual drugs with the same regimens in monotherapy for human-malaria are described below; and the PK data of five artemisinin drugs (AS, DHA, QHS, AM, and AE) corresponding with parasitological consequences in malaria patients are shown in **Table 1**, **Figures 1** and 2.

2.1 Intravenous-artesunate (IV-AS)

PK/PD profiles in humans were studied following AS intravenous administration at doses of 120 mg/person on the first day at 0 h followed by oral 100 mg at 8 h (**Figure 2**, top left). A mean peak level (C_{max}) of 11.343 ng/ml was displayed for IV-AS, which rapidly cleared with an elimination half-life of 0.05 h. The C_{max} of DHA, the primary metabolite of AS, was 2646 ng/ml with an elimination half-life

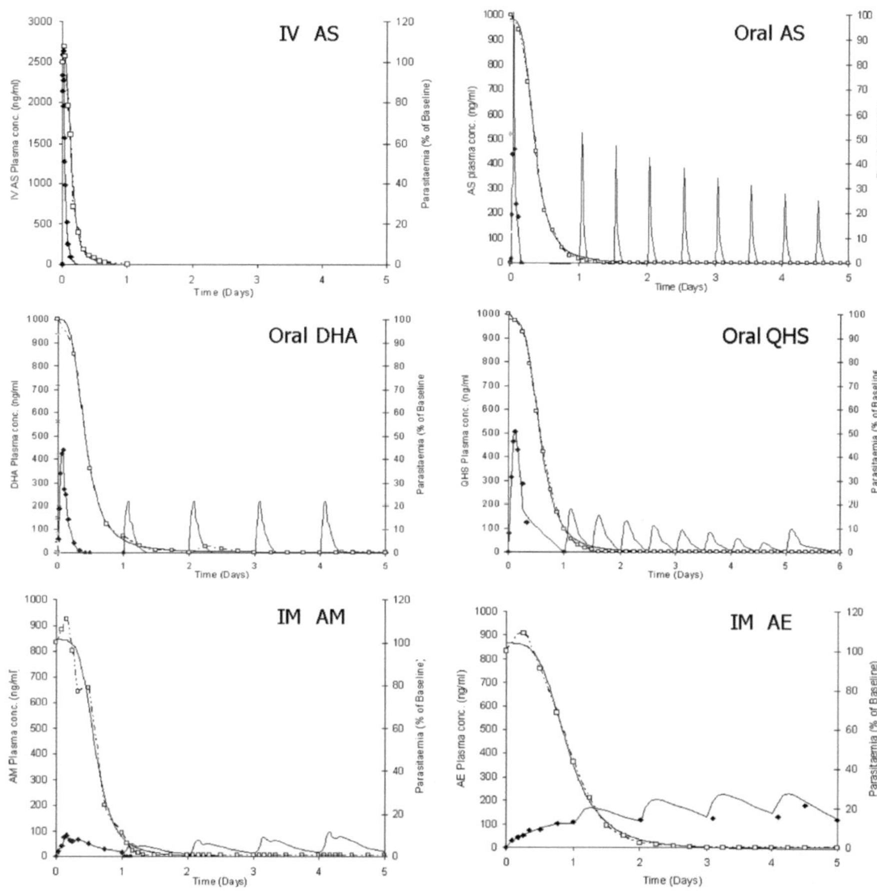

Figure 2.
Pharmacokinetic/pharmacodynamic profiles are in plasma following intravenous-artesunate and oral artesunate (AS, with DHA measurement) [22, 26–29], oral dihydroartemisinin (DHA) [30, 31], oral artemisinin (QHS) [19–21, 29], intramuscular artemether (AM) [35, 36], and arteether (AE) [38, 39] with various regimens measured by HPLC-ECD or LC-MS (solid markers) and computer-fitted curves (solid line) are from malaria human trials. Relative PK/PD parameters are given in **Table 1**, *and the parasitemia was counted 100% at zero while the first dosing time.*

of 0.67 h (**Table 1**). The mean AUC for DHA was 2378 ng h/ml, which is 2 times higher than that of the parent compound, AS, (AUC of 1146 ng h/ml) [26, 27].

In this trial, the lag phase for the parasitemia curve was estimated as 1.92 h (**Table 1**), which was the shortest as compared to oral AS and 4 other drugs (**Figure 1**, bottom), indicating that the IV-AS injection very efficiently kills parasites, with a mean time of 3.18 h for clearance of half the parasitemia (PC_{50}), which is the lowest PC_{50} and has the lowest area under inhibitory curve (AUIC) at 397.3% h/μl in this evaluation (**Table 1**). After modeling, an E_{max} of 0.00111% parasitemia was estimated for IV-AS therapy on the first day. The E_{max} was the principal pharmacodynamic parameter determining maximum antimalarial effects for the artemisinins, as it displayed a sharp concentration-effect relationships. This relationship may be due to the time that blood concentrations exceeded the minimum parasiticidal concentration (MPC), as opposed to being driven by either C_{max} or AUC [25]. For the data presented in this chapter, the MPC was the lowest after administration of100 mg per patient of IV-AS, with parasitemia remaining in blood (0.0011%) as compared to the other four artemisinin derivatives addressed (**Table 1**).

2.2 Oral artesunate (AS)

PK/PD profiles in plasma were studied following oral AS administration of 100 mg/person tablets on first day, followed by 50 mg twice daily for 2–6 days (**Figure 2**, top right). The mean peak plasma concentration of DHA was measured at 1052 ng/ml, with an elimination half-life of 0.75 h (**Table 1**). Also, the AS concentration declined day-over-day for the 5-day duration of dosing [22]. Mean AUC of DHA was calculated to be 1334 ng h/ml, 6.4 times higher than that of the parent compound (AUC of 210 ng h/ml), AS [28].

With the same oral dose regimen of AS, the time of lag phase in the parasitemia curve was only 2.81 h, shorter when compared to the four other artemisinins, with a range of 4.03–8.89 h (**Figure 1**, bottom) but longer than that of IV-AS (1.92 h), indicating that the effect of AS tablets was very efficient with a 0.36 h absorption half-life and a C_{max} of 1052 ng/ml [29]. Similarly, rapid parasite clearance with a mean time of 8.48 h for clearance of half the parasite load (PC_{50}), the lowest PC_{50} of the four drugs and the lowest AUIC with 921.2% h/μl (**Table 1**). After modeling, an E_{max} of 0.0016% parasitemia was calculated for oral treatment with AS on the first day. For the data presented here, the MPC was the lowest, with parasitemia remaining in blood after dosing with 100 mg of AS per patient as compared to other four artemisinin derivatives (**Table 1**).

2.3 Oral dihydroartemisinin (DHA)

Profiles of PK/PD in plasma following administration of 200 mg/person in tablets DHA on day 1 followed by 100 mg at day 2–5 are shown in **Figure 2** (middle left). After 200 mg of DHA, the mean peak plasma concentration of DHA was 437 ng/ml with an elimination half-life of 0.85 h. The mean AUC of DHA was calculated to be 1329 ng h/ml. With the 200 mg oral dose regimen, the time of lag phase in the parasitemia curve was 4.03 h, longer than that of oral (1.92 h) and IV-AS (2.81 h) but still shorter than either QHS (5.76 h), AM (7.26 h), or AE (8.89 h), indicating that the rapid clearance effect of DHA tablets was inferior to AS, but superior to QHS, AM, and AE regimens. Additionally, this rapid parasite clearance resulted in a mean time of 10.05 h of PC_{50} and an AUIC of 1167.9% h/μl (**Table 1, Figure 1**, bottom). After the first day, modeling estimates of the E_{max} were 0.213% parasitemia for oral DHA treatment. For the data presented here, after 200 mg per patient of DHA, high

MPC remained in the blood as compared to the other three artemisinin derivatives (**Table 1**). Absorption of DHA tablets, with 0.67 h half-life, was 50% slower than that of AS (0.36 h) in this trial as well, indicating that the relatively slow reduction of parasitemia may have resulted from the slow absorption [30, 31].

As compared to oral AS, the AUCs of treatments with either AS or DHA (in oral form) the same, with only C_{max} of oral AS differing, and was two times higher than oral DHA treatment, suggesting that this high peak concentration (C_{max}) may be causally related to the decrease of parasitemia in patients [30, 31]. DHA appeared to have very low bioavailability (<50%). If calculated with an equal dose level, the C_{max} and AUC_{DHA} estimated from AS treatment were four- and twofolds, respectively, higher than the DHA dosage regimen. Our data demonstrate that the DHA tablet (Cotexin) in beagle dogs had only 24.4% absolute bioavailability [32]. In malaria patients, rebound parasites (3%) on day 3 and one-fourth recrudescence rate (24%) were found in subjects treated with DHA tablets in clinical work [30]. The 3% of rebound parasites were only found in DHA oral treatment in this comparison (**Figure 2**).

2.4 Oral artemisinin (QHS)

PK/PD evaluation in plasma following artemisinin (QHS) oral administration of 500 mg/person on the first day followed by 250 mg twice daily for 4 days and then another 500 mg on 6th day is seen in **Figure 2** (middle right). After 500 mg of QHS by oral dosing, the mean peak plasma concentration of QHS was reached at 588 ng/ml and then declined with an elimination half-life calculated at 2.4 h. The mean AUC of QHS was estimated at 2601 ng h/ml, which was a comparatively high AUC due to the oral dose taken. With the 500 mg oral dosage regimen, the lag time in the parasitemia curve was 5.76 h, which was longer than oral and IV-AS (1.92–2.81 h) and DHA (4.03 h) but was better than AM and AE in trials (**Figure 1**, bottom). This indicates that the rapid effect of QHS capsules was not as good as oral AS and DHA even given at three- to sixfold higher doses [19–21, 29]. The patients treated with oral QHS showed 13.95 h of PC_{50} and the 1464.4% h/μl of AUIC (**Table 1**). The absorption of QHS capsules with a 1.21 h half-life was slower than the absorptions of AS and DHA drugs, suggesting that the slow reduction of parasitemia may have resulted from slow absorption and lower antimalarial potency. Compared with oral AS and DHA study, oral QHS appeared to have very low bioavailability of 30% [33] and low antimalarial potency with cultured *P. falciparum* [34].

2.5 Intramuscular artemether (AM)

PK and PD profiles in plasma following AM intramuscular administration in sesame oil of 3.2 mg/kg on day 1 and then 1.6 mg/kg daily on day 2–5 can be seen in **Figure 2** (bottom, left). The mean peak plasma concentration was reached at 74.9 ng/ml and then declined with an elimination half-life calculated at 7.83 h (**Table 1**), indicating that this formulation had the lowest peak of drug concentration when compared to the other four artemisinin drugs. A mean AUC was estimated at 1230 ng h/ml [35, 36]. At the same dosage regimen, the time of lag phase in the parasitemia curve was 7.26 h, which was the second longest lag time compared with the other three drugs except for AE, indicating that the effect of the AM intramuscular formulation had a very low and prolonged absorption from muscle injection sites [37].

Parasitemia counts early after dosing did not decrease due to the low peak concentration of AM, but increased markedly to 110% at 4 h (parasitemia was set at 100% of the zero dosing time). This observation may explain why the lag time was longer at 7.26 h with no parasite decrease after injection. Similarly, there was very slow clearance of parasites producing a mean PC_{50} time of 15.6 h (**Figure 1**, bottom), which was also the longest PC_{50} time compared to the other three drugs except AE (**Table 1**). The AUIC of 1613.4% h/μl also revealed that this drug given as an intramuscular regimen was not efficacious in reducing parasitemia [35]. Although intramuscular AM was not fast enough to kill parasites in patients, the long-lasting exposure level of AM (7.83 h elimination half-life) could reduce parasitemia at an acceptable rate. Computer modeling estimated the E_{max} at 0.003% parasitemia in this clinical trial. The MPC (E_{max}) was only a little more than oral AS in the first-day modeling, but much less than oral DHA, oral QHS, and intramuscular AE (**Table 1**).

2.6 Intramuscular arteether (AE)

PK and PD profiles in plasma following AE intramuscular administration in sesame oil of 4.8 mg/kg at 0 h and 1.6 mg/kg at 6 h on day 1 and then daily 1.6 mg from day 2–5 are illustrated in **Figure 2** (bottom, right). The mean peak plasma concentration was reached at 110.1 ng/ml and then declined with an elimination half-life calculated at 22.7 h (**Table 1**), indicating that this formulation has a low peak of drug concentration when compared to AS, DHA, and QHS. Mean AUC was estimated at 4702 ng h/ml [38]. At the same dosage, the lag time in the parasitemia curve was 8.89 h, which was the longest lag time and the highest AUC value compared with the other four drugs, indicating that the effect of the AE intramuscular formulation had a very low and prolonged absorption from muscle injection sites [37].

Parasitemia counts early after dosing did not decrease due to the low peak concentration of AE, but increased to 108% at 6 h (100% parasitemia set at 0 h of the first dosing time). As with AM, this increase may be the reason why the lag time is longer at 8.89 h with no parasite killing after injection. Similarly, a very slow parasite clearance was produced at mean PC_{50} time of 19.68 h, which was the longest PC_{50} time compared to the other four drugs (**Table 1**). The highest AUIC of 2463.5% h/μl revealed that the drug with the intramuscular regimen was not efficacious in reducing parasitemia [35, 39]. Intramuscular AE was neither able to exterminate parasites rapidly, nor to reduce parasitemia much in patients revealing it to be an inferior antimalarial agent when compared to the other four drugs (**Figure 1**, bottom). The computer modeling estimated the E_{max} at 0.55% parasitemia in this clinical trial. In spite of two doses on day 1 (4.8 mg/kg at 0 h and 1.6 mg/kg at 6 h), the E_{max} was still the highest value compared to other the four artemisinins (**Table 1**).

3. Efficacy and potency of artemisinins depending on drug peak concentration

Intravenous and oral AS are the fastest killers of parasites in human malaria treatments out of the five artemisinins, indicating that AS is a superior antimalarial agent in performance of PK/PD. IV-AS provides the highest peak concentration and a very short exposure time, while oral AS can also provide high peak levels and similar short exposure times. The data suggest that the higher peak level has a major role in eliminating parasites rapidly and the short exposure time contributes to the avoidance of fatal neurotoxicity [40, 41] as well as prevention of resistance [42].

Although DHA has similar efficacy to AS *in vitro* [34], the agent does not have as rapid effect as IV-AS or oral AS, even with twofold higher dosing. The explanations include lower bioavailability [43, 44], which results in a slower absorption phase, and a long lag time which has an effect on activity. However, we believe the principal reason is due to the lower peak concentration observed when compared to oral AS.

Oral artemisinin (QHS) does not compete well in this PK/PD comparison with its relatively low potency against cultured *P. falciparum* [34]. Although high oral doses (three- to sixfolds higher than oral DHA and AS, **Table 1**) produced higher plasma concentrations (2601 ng h/ml of AUC) and high peak concentrations (588 ng/ml), the relatively low potency [34] and bioavailability [33] significantly limited the efficacy.

Intramuscular AM or AE consistently displays low efficacy and slow parasite killing. Due to the sesame oil formulation, AM and AE have a very low and prolonged absorption from muscle injection sites [37]. Initially, parasitemia counts after dosing do not decrease due to the low and delayed peak concentrations (75–110 ng/ml) of AM and AE. This may be the main reason for slow elimination of parasites as the observed lag times of 7.2–8.9 h are the longest of the drugs. Subsequently, they have the slowest clearance rates, with mean PC_{50} times of 15.63–19.68 h, potentially resulting in inadmissible failures in some of the AE trials (**Table 1**) [38]. Although drug exposure times of AM and AE are comparatively longer than AS, DHA, and QHS, this long exposure apparently did not improve efficacy. Instead, it seems to induce neurotoxicity [41]; therefore, this formulation should not be encouraged for clinical use to treat acute and severe malaria as safer agents are available.

PK/PD evaluations demonstrate that the rapid efficacy of the artemisinins is principally due to the drug peak concentration (C_{max}). This further indicates that AS has superior PK/PD following either oral or intravenous administration. Other pharmacokinetic parameters, such as drug exposure level (AUC) and drug exposure time (half-life), tend to be of minor importance for efficacy [45]. Most clinical observations demonstrate that the fast pharmacodynamic properties of these drugs have been largely addressed with pharmacokinetic findings [38, 45, 46]. Further, low drug exposure of artemisinins may be a cause for observed treatment failures [37, 47, 48]. These studies showed that using a low dose regimen may not provide enough drug exposure to kill the parasites in these patients [49]. In contrast, the clinical cure indicated that the intravenous formulations, like AS injection, are very important in the rapid treatment of malaria with high observed peak concentrations (C_{max}), especially in severe and complicated malaria [26, 27].

Evidence shows that higher plasma concentrations (C_{max} and AUC), especially peak concentrations (C_{max}), greatly enhance the efficacy and clinical therapeutic potentials of the artemisinins. As previously discussed, the severity of the possible complications for *P. falciparum* malaria constitutes a serious medical emergency, and appropriate treatment should be initiated if infection is suspected. Appropriate treatment requires enough high-dose regimens and should be given to provide successful therapeutic efficacy for malaria patients, as it is known that 84% of all malaria related deaths occur within 24 h of hospital admission in African children [50]. As such, first exposure concentrations of artemisinin drugs are critical in the clinical setting.

4. PK/PD evaluation of artemisinin-based combination therapies (ACTs)

In order to avoid a high recrudescence of the monotherapy of artemisinins and to delay or prevent emergence of artemisinin resistance, WHO recommends the use of combination therapies for the treatment of uncomplicated *P. falciparum* malaria. Artemisinin derivatives rapidly decrease the parasite biomass, while the presence of partner antimalarial drugs with a different and slow-acting mechanism reduces the probability of high recrudescence. These therapies include one artemisinin derivative plus a partner, slow-acting, antimalarial drug with a longer half-life [51, 52].

WHO encourages the development of fixed-dose combination (FDC) versions of ACTs, versus coblistered tablets that can be misused to facilitate administration of artemisinin as monotherapy.

Two ACT combinations, artesunate-sulfadoxine/pyrimethamine (AS-SP) and artesunate-amodiaquine (AS-AQ), are used in areas where parasites are susceptible to these drugs. In areas where resistance to sulfonamide-pyrimethamine, chloroquine, and amodiaquine is prevalent, other artemisinin combinations are used such as artemether-lumefantrine (AL) or artesunate-mefloquine (AS-MQ). More recently, dihydroartemisinin-piperaquine (DP) is a promising ACT option that exhibits an excellent efficacy and safety profile and is currently the first-line therapy for uncomplicated malaria in Asia. Currently, artemisinins have been introduced to the market combined with other slow-acting drugs to create fixed-dose ACTs containing amodiaquine, mefloquine, and piperaquine [53].

Artemisinin-resistant *falciparum* malaria has developed on the border between Thailand and Cambodia. The development of artemisinin resistance is likely a consequence of patient treatment with artemisinin monotherapy with substandard, counterfeit, or adulterated drugs for over 40 years. This artemisinin resistance phenomenon is characterized clinically by much slower parasite clearance rates after artemisinin treatment [54]. This artemisinin resistance, defined by a delayed parasite clearance time, has been associated with several genetic mutations.

One hypothesis to explain this phenomenon is delayed parasite clearance derived from a stage-specific decrease in artemisinin sensitivity against circulating young asexual ring-stage parasites. Another hypothesis to explain this phenomenon is dormancy of ring-stage parasites *in vivo*, which would render them resistant to artemisinin treatment. A related hypothesis is that reduced sensitivity to treatment with artemisinins renders the ACT partner drug vulnerable to development of resistance. This very ominous development accompanied with the development of resistance over time in Asia to all of the partner drugs used for ACTs suggests that all of the current ACT regimens would be predicted to fail in Southeast Asia. This phenomenon will lead to malaria recurrence after treatment, and decreased efficacy of artemisinin-based treatment of severe malaria. To assess this question further concerning AS-MQ efficacy, a clinical trial was conducted on the Thai-Cambodian border using this combination to treat 151 subjects infected with uncomplicated *falciparum* malaria. Patients were followed over a 42 day period or until recurrent parasitemia was observed. The PCR-corrected treatment failure rate at 28 days was 13.1%, and the treatment failure rate at 42 days after treatment was 18.8%. These treatment failures were associated with longer parasite clearance times, increased *pfmdr1* copy number, increased initial parasitemia, and elevated mefloquine IC_{50} values. These data demonstrate the combined effects of artesunate resistance and mefloquine resistance in this region [55].

Similar to other drug resistance phenotypes, this resistance can best be understood based on its mechanism of action. More recently, it was demonstrated that artemisinin attacks multiple parasitic targets, suggesting that mutations in drug targets are unlikely to cause high-level artemisinin resistance. These findings will help us to better understand the mechanisms of artemisinin resistance and suggest that how can we continue to use ACTs [51].

There is a very large body of evidence to support the hypothesis that ACTs provide the best possible treatment available today for uncomplicated multidrug-resistant *falciparum* malaria. ACTs provide rapid treatment responses that are well tolerated, provide excellent cure rates with 3-day treatment regimens, provide reductions in gametocyte carriage, and decrease drug resistance by providing protection for combination partner drugs.

Clinical trials in 10 investigational sites in 7 African countries (Burkina Faso, Nigeria, Gabon, Zambia, Uganda, Rwanda, and Mozambique) were performed. About 4116 African children under 5 years of age with uncomplicated *P. falciparum* malaria were treated with four ACTs: 1226 with AL, 1002 with AS-AQ, 413 with chlorproguanil-dapsone-artesunate (CDA), and 1475 with DP. The PCR-corrected cure rate on day 63 showed no differences between DP, AL, and AS-AQ, while these three ACTs were statistically superior in comparison with CDA. The PCR-uncorrected cure rate at day 63 indicated that DP was statistically superior to AL, AS-AQ, and CDA [56].

In addition, the efficacy of the Eurartesim® formulation of DP in Thailand, Laos, and India was compared with that of AS-MQ for the treatment of patients aged 3 months to 65 years with uncomplicated *P. falciparum* malaria in a noninferiority trial conducted in Asia. DP was shown to be a highly efficacious drug for the treatment of uncomplicated *P. falciparum* malaria in areas where multidrug parasites are prevalent [57].

Several additional trials compared the efficacy of the Artekin® formulation of DP versus AS-MQ in patients with uncomplicated *P. falciparum* malaria. Most of the trials were conducted in Asia with one trial conducted in Peru, and the majority of trials included both pediatric and adult patients. DP was shown to be highly effective for the treatment of uncomplicated *P. falciparum* malaria [58].

Antimalarial drug resistance is now well established in both *P. falciparum* and *P. vivax*. In southern Papua, Indonesia, where both strains of *Plasmodia* coexist, a series of studies were conducted to optimize treatment strategies. A randomized trial compared the efficacy and safety of DP with AS-AQ. Of the 334 patients in the evaluable patient population, 185 were infected with *P. falciparum*, 80 were infected with *P. vivax*, and 69 were infected with both species. DP was both more efficacious and better tolerated than AS-AQ when used to treat multidrug-resistant *P. falciparum* and *P. vivax* infections. The prolonged therapeutic effects of piperaquine appeared to delay the time to *P. falciparum* reinfection, decrease the rate of recurrence of *P. vivax* infection, and reduce the risks of both gametocyte carriage and anemia [59].

Other studies have also shown that DP has excellent efficacy for the treatment of uncomplicated malaria. The results showed that DP was superior to AL and AS-AQ for reducing the risk of recurrent parasitemia and recrudescence [60]. DP has consistently been shown to be well tolerated, safe, and efficacious in adults and children in Asia, Africa, and South America, both in children and in adults with uncomplicated malaria due to *P. falciparum*, *P. vivax*, or mixed infections with significantly less nausea, vomiting, and dizziness than AS-MQ [58, 61]. DP was also better tolerated, with no clinically significant cardiovascular or metabolic effects [58].

Recently, nine trials compared the efficacy of Eurartesim®, Duocotecxin®, or Artekin® formulations of DP with that of AL in patients with uncomplicated *P. falciparum* malaria. Most of these trials were conducted in Africa, with one trial conducted in Cambodia. These additional trials demonstrated the efficacy of DP for the treatment of uncomplicated *P. falciparum* malaria. DP was shown to be superior to AL with respect to other endpoints, including fever and parasite clearance times, reinfection rates, and gametocyte carriage rates [58].

The conclusions of those studies were that DP was shown to be a safe, well tolerated, and highly effective treatment of *P. falciparum* malaria in Asia and Africa, but the effect on gametocyte carriage was inferior to that of AS-MQ [62].

5. Therapeutic effects of ACTs depending on the half-life of partner drug

Concerning therapeutic benefits, combination therapy minimizes the risk of emergence and spread of parasites resistant to either agent. Preventing the development of artemisinin resistance is of vital importance given the crucial role artemisinin derivatives play in malaria control and treatment programs. Artesunate resistance has already emerged in western Cambodia [1, 63]; however, ACTs are still capable of achieving cure rates exceeding 90%. Since 2001, WHO guidelines have recommended the use of ACTs to include DP, AL, AS-MQ, AS-AQ, and AS-SP to treat patients with uncomplicated *P. falciparum* malaria. Among those ACTs, DP represents a new and extremely promising fixed-dose combination. Several clinical trials have repeatedly shown that DP is a safe and highly efficacious therapy against uncomplicated *P. falciparum* and the asexual stages of *P. vivax* malaria. The risk of recurrent infections was significantly lower for DP, followed by AS-AQ and then AL, supporting the recent WHO recommendation to consider DP as a valid option for the treatment of uncomplicated *P. falciparum* malaria [64].

These therapies include one artemisinin derivative plus a partner compound, slow-acting, antimalarial drug with a longer half-life [51, 52]. The cumulative risk of parasitological failure was greater in studies of patients treated with AL, AS-MQ, and AS-SP than in patients treated with DP, reflecting the very long half-life of piperaquine. The long half-life of piperaquine is expected to have a major impact in improving the health-care systems of countries in *P. falciparum* malaria endemic areas (**Table 2**). Piperaquine has a large apparent volume of distribution (greater than 500 l/kg) and a terminal elimination half-life estimated around 5 weeks. With increasing sensitivity of assay techniques, the true terminal half-life is probably similar to that of chloroquine, 1–2 months. The oral bioavailability of piperaquine increases with coadministration with fat [58, 64–67].

In addition, the superior efficacy of DP for the treatment of *P. vivax* in malaria endemic areas versus chloroquine or other ACTs may reflect some measures of chloroquine resistance in areas where trials were conducted or comparison with one of the longer acting ACTs. Of the ACTs, DP has the longest half-life and as such was shown to be highly efficacious at preventing *P. vivax* relapses for up to 56 days following treatment. In a separate study, AS-MQ also provided protection against *P. vivax* parasitemia for up to 63 days. The shorter half-life combinations such as AL, although equally effective at rapidly reducing parasite biomass, were shown to provide comparatively little protection against early relapse [64–67]. Accordingly, the DP combination demonstrably has superior PK/PD qualities compared to all other ACTs recommended by WHO.

Antimalarials	Half-life of artemisinin derivative	Half-life of partner drug per full adult course (US$)	Regions currently in use purchase cost per course (US$)
Artemether-lumefantrine	~3 h	4–5 days	Africa, EM, SE Asia, WP and SA
Artesunate-mefloquine	<1 h	14–21 days	Africa, SE Asia, WP and SA
Artesunate-amodiaquine*	<1 h	9–18 days	Africa and EM
Dihydroartemisinin-	45 min	~5 weeks	Africa, SE Asia
piperaquine	<1 h	16 days	NA
Artesunate-pyronaridine	NA	1–2 months	Africa, EM, SE Asia, WP and SA
Chloroquine[1]	NA	~4 days (S) or	Africa, EM (IPT in Africa,
Sulfadoxine-pyrimethamine		~8 days (P)	EM and WP)

**This refers to the $t_{1/2}$ of the active metabolite monodesethylamodiaquine; the $t_{1/2}$ of amodiaquine is ~3 h*

[1]These former first-line antimalarials are included as a reference. EM, eastern Mediterranean; IPT, intermittent preventive treatment; NA, not applicable; P, pyrimethamine; S, sulfadoxine; SA, South America; SE Asia, Southeast Asia; $t_{1/2}$, half-life; WP, Western Pacific.

Table 2.
Plasma half-lives of the partner drugs used in artemisinin-based combination therapies (ACTs) [58, 64–67].

6. Conclusion

Artemisinins have been used clinically in the treatment of malaria for over 40 years, during which time their mechanism of action and pharmacokinetic properties have been elucidated. Empirical judgments concerning efficacy and optimal administration have been influenced by their impressive parasite clearance kinetics, which are superior to many commonly used alternatives. Among the five artemisinins in current use, the PK/PD profiles of AS are the best.

This report has also discussed the fact that the rapid efficacy of artemisinins is principally driven by peak concentration (C_{max}) from the first drug exposure. Other factors in the pharmacokinetic parameters, such as drug exposure level (AUC) and drug exposure time (half-life), appear to be of lesser importance. By the fundamental and reliable measures of efficacy in cure and mortality rates for uncomplicated and severe malaria, it is demonstrated that current artemisinins (AS, AM, and DHA), performing in roles as ACT or monotherapy, provide a clear-cut advantage over other antimalarials in some geographical locations. The most recent advances in the decrease of the mortality (34.7%) were shown with the use of IV-AS, as compared to IV quinine.

Although the artemisinins are poorly efficacious at achieving 100% cure in malaria when used as monotherapies, this shortage has been overcome using oral ACTs and IV-AS sequentially with a slower acting partner drug such as mefloquine or piperaquine. Previous arguments for the long-term benefits of combination and sequential therapies for preventing resistance and recrudescence still stand. The rapid action and subsequent decrease in mortality show that the artemisinins have a great advantage over other antimalarials when used as ACTs for uncomplicated malaria and in sequential therapy with AS injection in cases of severe and complicated malaria.

As a result of the long half-life of oral piperaquine, DP has excellent PK/PD potential when compared to all other ACTs. Importantly, WHO guidelines for the treatment of malaria expanded to include DP as an ACT option for the "first-line treatment of uncomplicated *P. falciparum* malaria worldwide" [53]. This was categorized as a "Strong Recommendation" and was added due to "High Quality Evidence."

Acknowledgements

This study was supported by the United States Army Research and Materiel Command. The opinions or assertions contained herein are the private views of the author and are not to be construed as official, or as reflecting true views of the Department of the Army or the Department of Defense.

Abbreviations

QHS	artemisinin
AS	artesunate
DHA	dihydroartemisinin
AE	arteether
AM	artemether
AL	artelinate
PK	pharmacokinetics
PD	pharmacodynamics

Author details

Qigui Li* and Brandon Pybus
Experimental Therapeutics Branch, Walter Reed Army Institute of Research, Silver Spring, Maryland, USA

*Address all correspondence to: qigui.li.civ@mail.mil

References

[1] Dondorp AM, Nosten F, Yi P, Das D, Phyo AP, Tarning J, et al. Artemisinin resistance in *Plasmodium falciparum* malaria. The New England Journal of Medicine. 2009;**361**:455-467. DOI: 10.1056/NEJMoa0808859

[2] Mathews ES, Odom John AR. Tackling resistance: Emerging antimalarials and new parasite targets in the era of elimination. F1000Research. 2018;7:pii: F1000. DOI: 10.12688/f1000research.14874.1

[3] Leang R, Taylor WR, Bouth DM, Song L, Tarning J, Char MC, et al. Evidence of *Plasmodium falciparum* malaria multidrug resistance to artemisinin and piperaquine in Western Cambodia: Dihydroartemisinin-piperaquine open-label multicenter clinical assessment. Antimicrobial Agents and Chemotherapy. 2015;**59**:4719-4726. DOI: 10.1128/AAC.00835-15

[4] Tyagi RK, Gleeson PJ, Arnold L, Tahar R, Prieur E, Decosterd L, et al. High-level artemisinin-resistance with quinine co-resistance emerges in *P. falciparum* malaria under in vivo artesunate pressure. BMC Medicine. 2018;**16**:181. DOI: 10.1186/s12916-018-1156-x

[5] Dondorp AM, Fairhurst RM, Slutsker L, Macarthur JR, Breman JG, Guerin PJ, et al. The threat of artemisinin-resistant malaria. The New England Journal of Medicine. 2011;**365**:1073-1075. DOI: 10.1056/NEJMp1108322

[6] Afaya A, Salia SM, Adatara P, Afaya RA, Suglo S, Japiong M. Patients' knowledge of artemisinin-based combination therapy treatment and its impact on patient adherence. Journal of Tropical Medicine. 2018;**2018**:7465254. DOI: 10.1155/2018/7465254

[7] White NJ. Delaying antimalarial drug resistance with combination chemotherapy. Parasitologia. 1999;**41**:301-308. PMID: 10697872

[8] Mutabingwa TK. Artemisinin-based combination therapies (ACTs): Best hope for malaria treatment but inaccessible to the needy! Acta Tropica. 2005;**95**:305-315. DOI: 10.1016/j.actatropica.2005.06.009

[9] Plewes K, Kingston HWF, Ghose A, Wattanakul T, Hassan MMU, Haider MS, et al. Acetaminophen as a renoprotective adjunctive treatment in patients with severe and moderately severe *falciparum* malaria: A randomized, controlled, open-label trial. Clinical Infectious Diseases. 2018;**67**:991-999. DOI: 10.1093/cid/ciy213

[10] Fanello C, Onyamboko M, Lee SJ, Woodrow C, Setaphan S, Chotivanich K, et al. Post-treatment haemolysis in African children with hyperparasitaemic *falciparum* malaria; a randomized comparison of artesunate and quinine. BMC Infectious Diseases. 2017;**17**:575. DOI: 10.1186/s12879-017-2678-0

[11] Whitty CJ, Ansah E, Reyburn H. Treating severe malaria. BMJ. 2005;**330**:317-318. DOI: 10.1136/bmj.330.7487.317

[12] Davis TM, Phuong HL, Ilett KF, Hung NC, Batty KT, Phuong VD, et al. Pharmacokinetics and pharmacodynamics of intravenous-artesunate in severe *falciparum* malaria. Antimicrobial Agents and Chemotherapy. 2001;**45**:181-186. DOI: 10.1128/AAC.45.1.181-186.2001

[13] Dondorp A, Nosten F, Stepniewska K, Day N, White N. South East Asian quinine artesunate malaria trial (SEAQUAMAT) group. Artesunate versus quinine for treatment of severe *falciparum* malaria: A randomised trial. Lancet. 2005;**366**:717-725. DOI: 10.1016/S0140-6736(05)67176-0

[14] Jelinek T. Intravenous-artesunate recommended for patients with severe malaria: Position statement from TropNetEurop. Euro Surveillance. 2005;**10**:E051124.5. PMID: 16794288

[15] Pasvol G. The treatment of complicated and severe malaria. British Medical Bulletin. 2006;**75-76**:29-47. DOI: 10.1093/bmb/ldh059

[16] Nosten F, Ashley E, McGready R, Price R. We still need artesunate monotherapy. BMJ. 2006;**333**:45. DOI: 10.1136/bmj.333.7557.45

[17] Li Q, Xie LH, Haeberle A, Zhang J, Weina P. The evaluation of radiolabeled artesunate on tissue distribution in rats and protein binding in humans. The American Journal of Tropical Medicine and Hygiene. 2006;**75**:817-826. PMID: 17123971

[18] Li Q, Xie LH, Johnson TO, Si YZ, Haeberle AS, Weina PJ. Toxicity evaluation of artesunate and artelinate in plasmodium berghei-infected and uninfected rats. Transactions of the Royal Society of Tropical Medicine and Hygiene. 2007;**101**:104-112. DOI: 10.1016/j.trstmh.2006.04.010

[19] Ashton M, Sy ND, Gordi T, Hai TN, Thach DC, Huong NV, et al. Evidence for time-dependence artemisinin kinetics in adults with uncomplicated malaria. Pharmaceutical and Pharmacological Letters. 1996;**6**:127-130

[20] van Agtmael MA, Cheng-Qi S, Qing JX, Mull R, van Boxtel CJ. Multiple dose pharmacokinetics of artemether in Chinese patients with uncomplicated *falciparum* malaria. International Journal of Antimicrobial Agents. 1999;**12**:151-158. PMID: 10418761

[21] Ashton M, Hai TN, Sy ND, Huong DX, Van Huong N, Nieu NT, et al. Artemisinin pharmacokinetics is time-dependent during repeated oral administration in healthy male adults. Drug Metabolism and Disposition. 1998;**26**:25-27. PMID: 9443848

[22] Khanh NX, de Vries PJ, Ha LD, van Boxtel CJ, Koopmans R, Kager PA. Declining concentrations of dihydroartemisinin in plasma during 5-day oral treatment with artesunate for *falciparum* malaria. Antimicrobial Agents and Chemotherapy. 1999;**43**:690-692. PMID: 10049291, PMCID: PMC89184

[23] Park BK, O'Neill PN, Maggs JL, Pirmohamed M. Safety assessment of peroxide antimalarials: Clinical and chemical perspectives. British Journal of Clinical Pharmacology. 1998;**46**:521-529. PMID: 9862239, PMCID: PMC1873802

[24] Le TA, Davis TM, Tran QB, Nguyen VP, Trinh KA. Delayed parasite clearance in a splenectomized patients with *falciparum* malaria who was treated with artemisinin derivatives. Clinical Infectious Diseases. 1997;**25**:923-925. PMID: 9356813

[25] White NJ. Clinical pharmacokinetics and pharmacodynamics of artemisinin and derivatives. Transactions of the Royal Society of Tropical Medicine and Hygiene. 1994;**88**:S41-S43. PMID: 8053024

[26] Batty KT, Thu LT, Davis TM, Ilett KF, Mai TX, Hung NC, et al. A pharmacokinetic and pharmacodynamic study of intravenous vs oral artesunate in uncomplicated *falciparum* malaria. British Journal of Clinical Pharmacology. 1998;**45**:123-129. PMID: 9491824, PMCID: PMC1873351

[27] Batty KT, Le AT, Ilett KF, Nguyen PT, Powell SM, Nguyen CH, et al. A pharmacokinetic and pharmacodynamic study of artesunate for vivax malaria. The American Journal of Tropical Medicine and Hygiene. 1998;**59**:823-827. PMID: 9840605

[28] Newton PN, Suputtamongkol Y, Teja-Isavadharm P, Pukrittayakamee S,

Navaratnam V, Bates I, et al. Antimalarial bioavailability and disposition of artesunate in acute *falciparum* malaria. Antimicrobial Agents and Chemotherapy. 2000;**44**:972-977. PMID: 10722499, PMCID: PMC89800

[29] Hassan Alin M, Ashton M, Kihamia CM, Mtey GJ, Bjorkman A. Multiple dose pharmacokinetics of oral artemisinin and comparison of its efficacy with that of oral artesunate in *falciparum* malaria patients. Transactions of the Royal Society of Tropical Medicine and Hygiene. 1996;**90**:61-65. PMID: 8730315

[30] Wilairatana P, Chanthavanich P, Singhasivanon P, Treeprasertsuk S, Krudsood S, Chalermrut K, et al. A comparison of three different dihydroartemisinin formulations for the treatment of acute uncomplicated *falciparum* malaria in Thailand. International Journal for Parasitology. 1998;**28**:1213-1218. PMID: 9762567

[31] Na-Bangchang K, Tippawangkosol P, Thanavibul A, Ubalee R, Karbwang J. Pharmacokinetic and pharmacodynamic interactions of mefloquine and dihydroartemisinin. International Journal of Clinical Pharmacology Research. 1999;**19**:9-17. PMID: 10450538

[32] Bennett K, Si Y, Steinbach T, Zhang J, Li Q. Pharmacokinetic and pharmacodynamic evaluation of intramuscular artesunate in healthy beagle dogs. The American Journal of Tropical Medicine and Hygiene. 2008;**79**:36-41. PMID: 18606761

[33] Koopmans R, Ha LD, Duc DD, Dien TK, Kager PA, Khanh NX, et al. The pharmacokinetics of artemisinin after administration of two different suppositories to healthy Vietnamese subjects. The American Journal of Tropical Medicine and Hygiene. 1999;**60**:244-247. PMID: 10072143

[34] Li Q, Gerena L, Xie L, Zhang J, Kyle D, Milhous W. Development and validation of flow cytometric measurement for parasitemia in cultures of *P. falciparum* vitally stained with YOYO-1. Cytometry. Part A. 2007;**71**:297-307. DOI: 10.1002/cyto.a.20380

[35] Murphy S, Watkins WM, Bray PG, Lowe B, Winstanley PA, Peshu N, et al. Parasite viability during treatment of severe *falciparum* malaria: Differential effects of artemether and quinine. The American Journal of Tropical Medicine and Hygiene. 1995;**53**:303-305. PMID: 7573718

[36] Aderibigbe BA. Design of drug delivery systems containing artemisinin and its derivatives. Molecules. 2017;**22**:pii: E323. DOI: 10.3390/molecules22020323

[37] Li Q, Brueckner RP, Peggins JO, Trotman KM, Brewer TG. Arteether toxicokinetics and pharmacokinetics in rats after 25 mg/kg/day single and multiple doses. European Journal of Drug Metabolism and Pharmacokinetics. 1999;**24**:213-223. PMID: 10716059

[38] Li Q, Lugt CB, Looareesuwan S, Krudsood S, Wilairatana P, Vannaphan S, et al. Pharmacokinetic investigation on the therapeutic potential of artemotil (beta-arteether) in Thai patients with severe *Plasmodium falciparum* malaria. The American Journal of Tropical Medicine and Hygiene. 2004;**71**:723-731. PMID: 15642961

[39] Looareesuwan S, Oosterhuis B, Schilizzi BM, Sollie FA, Wilairatana P, Krudsood S, et al. Dose-finding and efficacy study for i.m. Artemotil (beta-arteether) and comparison with i.m. Artemether in acute uncomplicated *P. falciparum* malaria. British Journal of Clinical Pharmacology. 2002;**53**:492-500. PMID: 11994055, PMC: 1874374

[40] Li Q, Mog SR, Si YZ, Kyle DE, Gettayacamin M, Milhous WK.

Neurotoxicity and efficacy of arteether related to its exposure times and exposure levels in rodents. The American Journal of Tropical Medicine and Hygiene. 2002;**66**:516-525. PMID: 12201585

[41] Li Q, Weina PJ. In: Li Q, Weina P, editors. Antimalarial in Drugs: Age of the Artemisinins. 1st ed. New York: Nova Science Publishers Inc; 2011. 645 p. ISBN-978-1-61761-851-2. Available from: https://books.google.com/books/about/Antimalarial_Drugs.html?id=hL5pngEACAAJ [Accessed: October 18, 2018]

[42] White NJ. Antimalarial drug resistance. The Journal of Clinical Investigation. 2004;**113**:1084-1092. PMID: 15085184, PMCID: PMC385418

[43] Binh TQ, Ilett KF, Batty KT, Davis TM, Hung NC, Powell SM, et al. Oral bioavailability of dihydroartemisinin in Vietnamese volunteers and in patients with *falciparum* malaria. British Journal of Clinical Pharmacology. 2001;**51**: 541-546. PMID: 11422013, PMCID: PMC2014487

[44] Na-Bangchang K, Krudsood S, Silachamroon U, Molunto P, Tasanor O, Chalermrut K, et al. The pharmacokinetics of oral dihydroartemisinin and artesunate in healthy Thai volunteers. The Southeast Asian Journal of Tropical Medicine and Public Health. 2004;**35**:575-582. PMID: 15689069

[45] Roussel C, Caumes E, Thellier M, Ndour PA, Buffet PA, Jauréguiberry S. Artesunate to treat severe malaria in travellers: Review of efficacy and safety and practical implications. Journal of Travel Medicine. 2017;**24**(2):1-9. DOI: 10.1093/jtm/taw093

[46] Kyle DE, Teja-Isavadharm P, Li Q, Leo K. Pharmacokinetics and pharmacodynamics of qinghaosu derivatives: How do they impact on the choice of drug and the dosage regimens? Medecine Tropicale: Revue du Corps de sante colonial. 1988;**58**(3 Suppl):38-44. PMID: 10212896

[47] Karbwang J, Na-Bangchang K, Thanavibul A, Molunto P. Plasma concentrations of artemether and its major plasma metabolite, dihydroartemisinin, following a 5-day regimen of oral artemether, in patients with uncomplicated *falciparum* malaria. Annals of Tropical Medicine and Parasitology. 1998;**92**:31-36. PMID: 9614451

[48] Silamut K, Newton PN, Teja-Isavadharm P, Suputtamongkol Y, Siriyanonda D, Rasameesoraj M, et al. Artemether bioavailability after oral or intramuscular administration in uncomplicated *falciparum* malaria. Antimicrobial Agents and Chemotherapy. 2003;**47**:3795-3798. PMID: 14638485, PMCID: PMC296187

[49] Sharma P, Swarup D, Saxena GN, Bhandari S, Sharma UB, Tuteja R. An open study to evaluate the efficacy of artemether in severe *falciparum* malaria. The Journal of the Association of Physicians of India. 1999;**47**:883-885. PMID: 10778657

[50] Shretta R, Liu J, Cotter C, Cohen J, Dolenz C, Makomva K, et al. Malaria elimination and eradication. In: Holmes KK, Bertozzi S, Bloom BR, Jha P, editors. Major Infectious Diseases, Chapter 12. 3rd ed. Washington, DC: The International Bank for Reconstruction and Development/The World Bank; 2017. PMID: 30212099

[51] Wang J, Xu C, Lun ZR, Meshnick SR. Unpacking 'Artemisinin resistance'. Trends in Pharmacological Sciences. 2017;**38**:506-511. DOI: 10.1016/j.tips.2017.03.007

[52] Eastman RT, Fidock DA. Artemisinin-based combination therapies: A vital tool in efforts to

eliminate malaria. Nature Reviews. Microbiology. 2009;7:864-874. DOI: 10.1038/nrmicro2239

[53] WHO. Guidelines for the Treatment of Malaria. 3rd ed. Geneva: World Health Organization; 2015. Available from: http://www.who.int/malaria/publications/atoz/9789241549127/en/ [Accessed: October 15, 2018]

[54] Dondorp AM, Yeung S, White L, et al. Artemisinin resistance: Current status and scenarios for containment. Nature Reviews. Microbiology. 2010;**8**:272-280. DOI: 10.1038/nrmicro2331.

[55] Rogers WO, Sem R, Tero T, Chim P, Lim P, Muth S, et al. Failure of artesunate-mefloquine combination therapy for uncomplicated *Plasmodium falciparum* malaria in southern Cambodia. Malaria Journal. 2009;**8**:10. DOI: 10.1186/1475-2875-8-10

[56] Sigma-Tau. Application for Inclusion of Dihydroartemisinin Plus Piperaquine (DHA/PPQ) Fixed Dose Combination Tablets in the 17th edition of the WHO Model Lists of Essential Medicines. Available from: http://www.who.int/selection_medicines/committees/expert/18/applications/D_Piperaquine.pdf [Accessed: October 15, 2018]

[57] Valecha N, Phyo AP, Mayxay M, Newton PN, Krudsood S, Keomany S, et al. An open-label, randomised study of dihydroartemisinin-piperaquine versus artesunate-mefloquine for *falciparum* malaria in Asia. PLoS One. 2010;**5**:e11880. DOI: 10.1371/journal.pone.0011880

[58] Keating GM. Dihydroartemisinin/piperaquine: A review of its use in the treatment of uncomplicated *Plasmodium falciparum* malaria. Drugs. 2012;**72**:937-961. DOI: 10.2165/11203910-000000000-00000

[59] Hasugian AR, Purba HL, Kenangalem E, Wuwung RM, Ebsworth EP, Maristela R, et al. Dihydroartemisinin-piperaquine versus artesunate-amodiaquine: Superior efficacy and posttreatment prophylaxis against multidrug-resistant *Plasmodium falciparum* and plasmodium vivax malaria. Clinical Infectious Diseases. 2007;**44**:1067-1074. DOI: 10.1086/512677

[60] Yeka A, Harris JC. Treating uncomplicated malaria in children: Comparing artemisinin-based combination therapies. Current Opinion in Pediatrics. 2010;**22**:798-803. DOI: 10.1097/MOP.0b013e32833fac44

[61] D'Alessandro U. Progress in the development of piperaquine combinations for the treatment of malaria. Current Opinion in Infectious Diseases. 2009;**22**:588-592. DOI: 10.1097/QCO.0b013e328332674a

[62] Zwang J, Ashley EA, Karema C, D'Alessandro U, Smithuis F, Dorsey G, et al. Safety and efficacy of dihydroartemisinin-piperaquine in *falciparum* malaria: A prospective multi-Centre individual patient data analysis. PLoS One. 2009;**4**:e6358. DOI: 10.1371/journal.pone.0006358

[63] Ariey F, Witkowski B, Amaratunga C, Beghain J, Langlois AC, Khim N, et al. A molecular marker of artemisinin-resistant *Plasmodium falciparum* malaria. Nature. 2014;**505**:50-55. DOI: 10.1038/nature12876

[64] Sousa M, Pozniak A, Boffito M. Pharmacokinetics and pharmacodynamics of drug interactions involving rifampicin, rifabutin and antimalarial drugs. The Journal of Antimicrobial Chemotherapy. 2008;**62**:872-878. DOI: 10.1093/jac/dkn330

[65] Sinclair D, Gogtay N, Brand F, Olliaro P. Artemisinin-based combination therapy for treating uncomplicated plasmodium vivax malaria. Cochrane

Database of Systematic Reviews. 2011;(7):CD008492. DOI: 10.1002/14651858.CD008492.pub2

[66] Bassat Q. The use of artemether-lumefantrine for the treatment of uncomplicated plasmodium vivax malaria. PLoS Neglected Tropical Diseases. 2011;**5**:e1325. DOI: 10.1371/journal.pntd.0001325

[67] Douglas NM, Anstey NM, Angus BJ, Nosten F, Price RN. Artemisinin combination therapy for vivax malaria. The Lancet Infectious Diseases. 2010;**10**:405-416. DOI: 10.1016/S1473-3099(10)70079-7

Chapter 5

Nipping the Malaria Vectors in the Bud: Focus on Nigeria

Omolade Olayinka Okwa

Abstract

Vector control is an important component of malaria control. Human malaria is a mosquito-borne parasitic disease which causes up to a million deaths a year and is estimated to infect over 212 million people worldwide. It is present in 97 countries covering half of the world's population. Around 90% of deaths occur in sub-Saharan Africa, especially Nigeria and the Democratic Republic of the Congo (DRC). Malaria is the most widespread mosquito-borne disease in Nigeria where it has a holoendemic status. Of the four malaria parasites in Africa, *Plasmodium falciparum* is the most common malaria species, while *Anopheles gambiae sensu stricto* is the predominant vector in Nigeria. This review discusses the challenges to control malaria in Nigeria which gives a larger picture of sub-Saharan Africa. These challenges include the adaptability of the anopheles mosquito to the environment, their diversity, and their different vectorial capacities. Despite all the efforts to control malaria, it is still a public health challenge in Nigeria and in sub-Saharan Africa. However, one of the basic challenges is the source which are the diverse breeding sites. This problem is enhanced by malariogenic activities of humans. Salient recommendations for vector control by nipping the malaria vector in the bud were identified and advocated.

Keywords: *Anopheles*, malaria, *Plasmodium*, vectors, Nigeria

1. Introduction

Human malaria is a parasitic disease caused by five species of *Plasmodium* (a protozoon) such as *P. falciparum*, *P. ovale*, *P. malariae*, *P. vivax*, and the zoonotic *P. knowlesi* in Asia. Globally, malaria causes up to a million deaths a year and is estimated to infect over 212 million people. It is present in 97 countries covering half of the world's population [1]. Around 90% of deaths occur in sub-Saharan Africa, especially in Nigeria and the Democratic Republic of the Congo (DRC) [2]. It is an established fact that malaria kills over a million children every year in sub-Saharan Africa [1, 3].

As a vector-borne disease, malaria vector control is an important component of malaria control. The malaria parasite has a complex life cycle, having a series of stages in the mosquito and the human host. The transmission of malaria takes place when the parasite enters the host through the saliva of the insect during a blood meal. As mosquitoes continue to threaten human health and existence, there is a need to continually fight back by nipping the malaria vectors in the bud by diverse mosquito control methods.

These concerns necessitate preventive approaches to control malaria by mosquito control methods that involve "nipping in the bud" from the source of the malaria problem.

IntechOpen

2. Mosquitoes as deadly insect vectors

Mosquitoes are slender, fragile, flying insects of about 3–6 mm in the order Diptera (true flies) within the invertebrate super-phylum Arthropoda. These insects are the deadliest animals on the planet earth, transmitting not only malaria parasites but also filariasis, yellow fever, dengue fever, Zika virus, Mayaro virus, Ross River virus, West Nile virus, Rift Valley fever, Japanese encephalitis, St. Louis encephalitis, chikungunya, and other pathogens and bringing death and misery to millions every year [4]. There are about 40 mosquito genera, and Africa is the home to three important, efficient, and deadly mosquito genera which are *Anopheles*, *Culex*, and *Aedes* species [5]. The female *Anopheles* belonging to one of these deadly genera transmits malaria even more than wild fire!

3. The adaptability of the *Anopheles* mosquitoes

Malaria is a problem in the tropics and not in temperate regions of the world. In the temperate countries, there are mosquitoes, but the life of the malaria parasite inside the mosquito is a race against time. The time taken for the malaria parasite to go through its growth and development is close to the average life span of the mosquito itself. This period is longer in the temperate areas where the survival of the parasite is on the knife edge, and temperature below certain point reduces the life span of the mosquito before it can transmit malaria [6].

The adaptability of *Anopheles* mosquitoes in the tropics and the ability to thrive in variety of habitats are a big challenge, and this is tantamount to greater spread of malaria.

Mosquitoes naturally infest ponds, marshes, puddles, swamps, and other wetland habitats. However, mosquitoes can also breed in any collection of still or stagnant waters [7].

Adult female mosquitoes may live up to a month in extreme cases in captivity but up to 2 weeks in nature. They are poikilothermic and have amazing adaptability such as suctorial mouthparts, holometabolous life cycle, and great diversity which are some of the secrets behind their success [8].

Both male and female *Anophele*s mosquitoes feed on sugary and plant juices as source of energy, flight, and dispersal. However, only the female mosquitoes feed on blood which is required every 2–3 days for the maturation of its eggs as the plant sources are inefficient. This blood sucking instinct is a mandatory biological process [9]. Female mosquitoes mate once in a lifetime and require still waters to oviposit. Mosquito goes through four stages during its life cycle. The first three stages egg, larva, and pupa are aquatic, but the adult is aerodynamic but may also rest on vegetation. More so, in Africa, malaria-carrying mosquitoes typically bite between dusk and dawn which coincides with the sleeping patterns of the people [3, 6].

3.1 The environment and the human malaria vectors

Distribution and incidence of vector-borne diseases are determined by the ecological conditions that favours them [10]. There is a relationship between the environment and mosquito abundance [11]. There are evidences that mosquito can adapt to environmental changes and even water pollution [12]. Today's mosquito breeds even where we thought they can never thrive due to environmental changes [9]. It has been established that climatic factors have profound influences on mosquito's life span [13]. As ecosystems are being modified across the planet, the habitat is altered, and malaria territories are being extended because of global warming.

Consequently, any small variations in microclimate can affect the mosquito's chances of survival or longevity [14].

3.1.1 Environmental factors

These include factors such as temperature, rainfall and humidity which are important factors for mosquito development, and longevity [15]. Changes in the local environment are important as they create or reduce the number of suitable breeding sites for vectors, so affecting their abundance and transmission pattern [16]. Temporal and spatial changes in temperature, precipitation, and humidity under different climatic conditions will affect the biology and ecology of malaria vectors and consequently the risk of malaria transmission [15].

3.1.2 Temperature

This factor has been regarded to be the most important factor affecting mosquitoes [17, 18]. A drop in temperature can change a mosquito's life span by more than 1 week. Small changes in temperature result in large differences in availability and development of mosquitoes. This implies that if temperature rises, the larvae takes a shorter time to mature and more offspring are produced. In fact, temperature affects metamorphic changes of mosquitoes in their breeding water sites [18]. This also means that the frequency of sucking and digesting of blood meal by female mosquitoes increases, and this has grave implications for malaria transmission [17].

3.1.3 Rainfall

This factor also plays a role in mosquito ecology as it increases the availability of surface water and so more breeding sites and affects relative humidity and hence longevity of the adult mosquito [6]. There is relatively lower temperature but higher relative humidity. Biting intensity of mosquito reduces as rainfall reduces and can be suspended at low temperature. Rainfall also determines the type of predominant malaria vector species. For example, *An. arabiensis* prevails in the dry season, while *An. gambiae sensu stricto* (ss) is a rainy season vector [8, 9].

3.1.4 Vegetation

Mosquitoes will rest in houses after feeding if there is no outdoor resting site. Vegetation increases outdoor resting sites and mosquito abundance, and type of species could relate to type of vegetation cover [19]. For example, it has been reported that *Anopheles arabiensis,* a malaria vector in Nigeria, predominates in the arid savanna, while *An. gambiae ss* is a forest-loving vector. *An. arabiensis* has been identified in deforested areas within forested areas in urban areas [6, 9].

4. The challenges of malaria vector control in Nigeria

4.1 Human malaria in Nigeria

Malaria is the most widespread mosquito-borne disease in Nigeria where it has a holoendemic status, the most vulnerable groups being children aged 0–5 years and pregnant women [3]. The disease accounts for 25% of infant mortality and 30% of childhood mortality [2]. Nigeria contributes the highest burden to global malaria morbidity and deaths. This is about 25% of global malaria cases, about 30% of global malaria deaths [20]. Malaria is one of the greatest causes of outpatient visits and work and school absenteeism in Nigeria [21, 22]. It has a familiar reputation of causing fever, headache, and teeth chattering shills and shakes [22]. Malaria is the number one killer disease in Nigeria where unfortunately, it is called "common" malaria. This is an irony! Malaria death has been described by an expert as causing death more than the deaths due to the first and second world wars [9]. No wonder the World Health Organization described mosquitoes as the deadliest animals on the planet earth [4].

P. falciparum is the most virulent species of malaria parasite in Nigeria. It causes 95% of infections, while *P. malariae* causes 5% of infections in Nigeria [23]. *P. ovale* is rarely seen, while *P. vivax* is absent in the whole of West Africa [24]. The risk of malaria exists throughout the country where it is a disease of public health concern. Malaria imposes immense morbidity and mortality as well as socioeconomic burdens on both individuals and the nation at large [21, 22].

4.2 Efforts to control human malaria in Nigeria

Nigeria is a large country and the most populous country in Africa (169 million; Nigeria population commission) and one of the hardest hit by malaria in the entire globe [25].

The Nigeria Federal Ministry of Health reported that Nigeria loses about 1.1 trillion naira annually to control malaria. A lot of funds have been invested on malaria drugs, insecticides, and mosquito nets for control of malaria. The Nigerian Minister of Health claimed that malaria reduces the country's gross domestic product (GDP) by 1% annually [26].

The burden of malaria in Nigeria is being managed through effective case management and vector control measures, including the use of insecticide-treated bed nets (ITNs) and indoor residual spraying (IRS). ITNs are now distributed freely to vulnerable groups in Nigeria. IRS is also one of the major vector control interventions used in Nigeria today. However, these methods have limitations in their usage [27].

Vector control has proven record in the prevention and control of vector-borne diseases. However, it is bad news that despite all the efforts to control mosquitoes in Nigeria, they are not even threatened or on the verge of extinction [9]. Malaria still remains a deadly scourge and formidable foe of public health concern. These are the main challenges:

4.3 Diverse anopheles species complexes and sibling species

Malaria transmission dynamics is a complex system that is superficially understood. For example, one has to deal with diversity of mosquito species in the tropics. The *An. gambiae* complex is the predominant vector in sub-Saharan Africa, but it is not the only vector in the field [18, 23].

- The *Anopheles gambiae* species complex consists of at least eight different sibling species: *An. gambiae (ss), An. arabiensis*, *An. melas*, *An. merus*, *An. quadrimaculatus A*, *An. quadrimaculatus B*, *An.bwambae*, *and An. coluzzi* [9, 23, 28].

- *An. funestus* species complex is another group of mosquitoes that play significant role in malaria transmission in sub-Saharan Africa. This complex occurs in sympatry with the *An. gambiae* complex [23, 29]. The eight sibling species of the *An. funestus* species complex are *An. funestus* ss, *An. rivulorum*, *An. vaneedi*, *An. leesoni*, *An. parensis*, *An. brucei*, *An. confuscus*, and *An. aruni*.

An. funestus ss like *An. gambiae ss* is also very widespread, highly endophilic, and anthropophilic and hence anthropophagic. Both complexes are polymorphic, biologically and genetically. Evidences suggest that they may share the same habitat, although *An. funestus ss* is more restricted in habitat choice than *An. gambiae ss* [18, 23, 30].

The behavior of each of the sibling species in both complexes varies and so their roles in malaria transmission. Hence, targeting only one sibling species by whatever method is not going to curb the menace of malaria. The diversity of the epidemiological situations within sub-Saharan ecotypes presents different malaria situation [31]. Comprehensive knowledge of behavior and heterogeneities that exist within, and among these vectors, will always be of benefit. Any strategy aiming at control will have to account for this heterogeneity in species diversity [32].

Malaria transmission dynamics is variable throughout Africa with huge variability in transmission patterns even within villages few kilometers apart [33]. The correct analysis of the distribution of specific malaria vectors is one of the prerequisites for meaningful epidemiological studies and for planning and monitoring of successful malaria control or eradication program [34].

In the past, large areas of Nigeria had no reliable data in the past on presence and absence of vectors [23]. It has been established that there are diversities of malaria vectors in Nigeria and they have different bionomics and vector competences. In Nigeria today, 35 *Anopheles* species have so far been recognized, but they do not all transmit malaria under the same circumstances. Some *Anopheles* mosquito species have unknown vector status, while some are non-malaria vectors ([9, 12]. However, the malaria transmission dynamics in Nigeria is mainly vectored by members of the *An. gambiae* complex such as *An. gambiae ss*, *An. coluzzi*, and *An. arabiensis*. *An .funestus ss* is also an important main vector, while *An. nili*, *An. melas*, and *An. moucheti* are localized vectors in Nigeria [9, 23, 29]. Secondary vectors in Nigeria include *An. pharoensis*, *An. coustani*, *An. hancocki*, and *An. longipalpis* [9, 12].

Control measures can only be effective if the abundance, behavior, and proportion of the vectors are known. The existence of species complexes containing morphologically cryptic sibling or isomorphic forms presents a major challenge to malaria control program as these require vector identification using molecular techniques [32].

Failure to know which sibling species one is dealing with will result in wasting scare resources and time to control non-malaria vectors [9].

4.4 Vectorial capacity and vectorial competence of the malaria vectors

The malaria problem in sub-Saharan Africa represents a peculiar case because the vectorial system is the most complex anywhere. This vectorial system diversity absolutely impacts malaria epidemiology and control [35].

Vectorial capacity and vectorial competence have been used interchangeably to describe the ability of mosquitoes to serve as a disease vector. The two terms are not synonyms because vectorial capacity is qualitative and is influenced by such variables as vector density, longevity, and vector competence itself [3]. Vectorial capacity takes into account environmental, behavioral, and cellular and biochemical factors that influence the association between a vector, the pathogen transmitted by the vector, and the host to which the pathogen is being transmitted [36].

However, vectorial competence is a component of vectorial capacity which is governed by intrinsic and generic factors that influence the ability of a vector to transmit a pathogen. For example, the susceptibility of an *Anopheles* mosquito to sporozoite stage of *Plasmodium* species is an important component of vectorial competence [37]. Vector competence, however, differs from one species to another and from place to place. There are *Anopheles* species complexes that vary in their behaviors, vectorial competences, and capacities, and these present a real problem to malaria control in the tropics [35].

The main factor governing the ability of *Anopheles* species to act as malaria vector is the frequency with which it feeds on humans [37]. These malaria vectors associated with stable malaria are those which are strongly antropophagic, often feeding on humans to the exclusion of other hosts. Anopheline vectors of malaria consist of various behaviors associated with their biting activities and hence transmission dynamics [38].

4.5 Malariogenic activities and lifestyles of humans

Malariogenic activities and lifestyles are human activities that promote the transmission of malaria. The ability of mosquitoes to thrive even outside their natural habitat makes them a nuisance to mankind. Man and environment are created to interact with each other on a balance basis, but man has failed in his duty to the environment. The responsibility of man is to respect, protect, and care for the environment [9, 12].

By sheer negligence, mosquito breeds just under our nose, right inside our homes, so house spraying and screening are obviously inadequate. People store water in containers in their homes because of poor water supply, being ignorant of the consequences.

In residential areas, human activities create mosquito breeding sites such as discarded trash cans, open buckets, clogged gutters, abandoned vehicles, tires, drainages, ditches, natural depressions, or just anywhere that can retain water. Inside homes, endophilic female mosquitoes rest in dark places, corners of rooms, and behind curtains, but the exophilic biters rest on vegetation after feeding. When the eggs are about to be laid, they go into any suitable water within and outside the houses to oviposit.

4.6 Diverse breeding sites of the anopheles mosquito

It will be cost-effective to deal with mosquitoes by "nipping them in the bud" through eliminating their very source. The remote source of the malaria problem in the tropics is the mosquito's adaptability to environmental conditions and diversity and indiscriminate types of breeding sites which are of great importance [16]. The crux of the matter is that the intricacy of mosquitoes extends even into their breeding sites [9].

There is a considerable paucity of adequate information regarding vector oviposition habits, where *Anopheles* rest during the day and in their preferred breeding sites [39].

This information is critical for control efforts as we will not need to bother too much on the species or sibling species type or their vectorial capacities.

However, most researchers do not take into account the menace of mosquito breeding sites and the attendant environmental factors. The source of mosquito problem can be just near you or about anywhere where stagnant or still water collects or is stored in homes. This should be appropriately incorporated into vector control program.

5. Recommendations for action

- Integrated management approach has been said to be the best for malaria control program, but they must take into account the breeding sites of mosquitoes.

- Knowledge, attitude, and practices (KAP) is the educational diagnosis of a community and is also essential for control program.
- Health and environmental education of the populace on preventing domestic mosquito breeding is essential. The following steps should be noted.
- Objects, excavations, plants, and anything that can hold water must be eliminated. Water storage containers in homes should always be covered.
- People should dispose unused containers and place useful ones upside down under a roof or seal with a tight cover.
- People must change frequently the water troughs of domestic and pet animals and garden flower pots around homes.
- People should keep trash cans tightly sealed and drill a hole at the bottom in order not to retain water that may serve as breeding sites.
- People should fill up eroded soils, natural depressions, and excavations and empty rain-filled receptacles. Swimming pools in homes should not be left unused and untreated.
- Outdoor spraying of domestic animal shelters, garages, outdoor latrines, and tree hole fillings must be carried out regularly.
- People should spray oil on stagnant pools around them to kill mosquito aquatic stages.
- Drainage system, ditches, and gutters must not be dumped with waste to avoid clogging, thereby making them stagnant for mosquitoes to breed.
- People should take action to prevent sewage effluents, soakaway, domestic run-offs and empty soft drink bottles from becoming breeding sites of mosquitoes.
- People should adhere to basic architectural designs; house designs with excavations or rain-filled receptacles should be discouraged such as the eave tube technology in Benue State, Nigeria [40]
- Environmental sanitation should be everybody's business. Enforcement of environmental sanitation by clearing bushes, cleaning drainages and open gutters, destruction and removal of containers, plants, tires, sachets, and anything that can hold water around homes will go a long way. Therefore education of the populace on mosquito breeding sites in homes is advocated.

6. Conclusion

No doubt, human malaria affects the health, wealth, and welfare of human populations.

The disease causes serious morbidity, human suffering, and mortality. These adverse consequences have led to increased need to wage a continuous war against malaria vectors by prevention not only at the local, national, and global levels but also at the domestic level.

Malariologists and vector biologists will benefit tremendously if the source of mosquito breeding sites is located and destroyed. This will reduce the transmission threshold of malaria to a considerable level. Malaria will not be readily controlled if we continue to ignorantly breed mosquitoes domestically.

Health education, the principle by which individuals and groups of people learn to behave in a manner conducive to the promotion, maintenance, or restoration of health, is applicable to malaria control. It not only teaches prevention and basic health knowledge but also conditions ideas that reshape everyday habits of people with unhealthy lifestyles in developing countries. This type of conditioning not only affects the immediate recipients of such education, but it also impacts the future generations who will benefit from improved and properly cultivated ideas about health that will eventually be ingrained with a ripple effect.

Acknowledgements

I thank Intech for the invitation to contribute this book chapter.

Conflict of interest

The author confirms that there is no conflict of interest.

Author details

Omolade Olayinka Okwa
Department of Zoology and Environmental Biology, Faculty of Science,
Lagos State University, Lagos, Nigeria

*Address all correspondence to: okwaomolade@hotmail.com

References

[1] WHO. World Malaria Report. Geneva: World Health Organization; 2013. 284 p. ISBN: 978 924 154694

[2] WHO. Global Burden of Diseases: 2004 Update. Geneva: World Health Organization; 2008. 160 p. ISBN: 978 924 1563710

[3] Okwa OO. Malaria, a pending problem in sub-Saharan Africa. In: Okwa O, editor. Malaria Parasites. Rijeka, Croatia: In-Tech Open Access Publisher; 2012. 350 p

[4] WHO. Global Strategy for Dengue Prevention and Control. Geneva: World Health Organization; 2015. 43 p. ISBN: 978 924 1504034

[5] WHO. World Malaria Report. Geneva: World Health Organization; 2014. 242 p. ISBN: 978 924 1564830

[6] Osta FM, Burket TR, Andre RJ. Behavioral aspects of mosquito. *Annual Revision of Entomology*. 2004;**34**: 401-421

[7] WHO. The African Malaria Report. Geneva, Switzerland: World Health Organization; 2006. 11 p

[8] Gillet JD. Common Africa Mosquitoes and Their Medical Importance. London: William Heinmann Medical Books, Limited; 1972

[9] Awolola TS. Malaria, Mosquitoes and Man: The Battle Continues! Nigeria Institute of Medical Research (NIMR): Distinguished Lecture Series. 7th ed. 2017. 73 p

[10] Marta FM. Impact of insecticide treated nets protecting cattle in zero-grazing units in nuisance and biting insects in the forest region of Kumasi, Ghana [Ph.D. thesis]. Institute of Parasitology and Tropical Veterinary Medicine, Free University of Berlin, Germany; 2009. 1SBN: 978-3-86664-643-8

[11] Chapman HC. Biological control of mosquitoes. Tropical Medicine and International Health. 2000;**10**:888-893

[12] Awolola TS, Oduola AO, Obansa JB, Chukwura NJ, Unyimordu JP. *Anopheles gambiae* breeding in polluted water in urban Lagos, south western Nigeria. Journal of Vector Borne Diseases. 2007;**44**:181-888

[13] Amerasinghe FP, Indrajith NG, Ariyasena TG. Physicochemical characteristics of mosquitoes breeding habitats in an irrigation development area in Sri-Lanka. Ceylon Journal of Medical Science (Biological Sciences). 1995;**24**(2):13-29

[14] Okorie TG. The breeding sites preferences of mosquitoes in Ibadan, Oyo state, Nigeria. Nigeria Journal of Entomology. 1978;**1**(3):71-80

[15] Becker N, Petrič D, Zgomba M, Boase C, Madon M, Dahl C. Mosquitoes and Their Control. 2nd ed. Heidelberg, Germany: Springer; 2010

[16] Beck-Johnson LM, Nelson WA, Paaijmans KP, Read AF, Thomas MB, Ornstard ON. The effect of temperature on *Anopheles* mosquito dynamics and potential for malaria transmission. PLoS One. 2013;**8**:79276

[17] Howlett F. The influence of temperature upon the biting of mosquitoes. Parasitology. 1910;**3**(4):479-481. DOI: 10.1017/ Soo31182000002304

[18] Kelly-Hope LA, Hemingway J, Mackenzie FE. Environmental factors associated with malaria vectors *Anopheles gambiae* and *Anopheles funestus* in Kenya. Malaria Journal. 2008;**8**:268

[19] Okogun GRA, Nwoke BEB, Okere AN, Anosike JC, Esekhegbe AC. Epidemiological implications of preferences of breeding sites of mosquito species in Mid- western Nigeria. Annual Agricultural and Environmental Medicine. 2013;**10**:217-222

[20] Arowolo T. Ending Malaria in Nigeria: The WHO Agenda: Paper Presented at Nigerian Institute of Medical Research, Yaba, Lagos, Nigeria on the World Malaria Day; 27 April 2016

[21] Okwa OO, Bello BA, Olundegun SA. Social aspects of malaria in two tertiary institutions in Lagos state, Nigeria. Sierra Leone Journal of Biomedical. Research. 2011;**3**(2):97-103. ISSN online: 2219-3170

[22] Okwa OO, Sanyaolu LO, Olatokunbo AF. Malaria and working performances of academic staff in a Nigerian University. Research Journal of Biology. 2012;**2**(5):151-156. ISSN: 2049-1727

[23] Okwa OO, Akinmolayan IF, Carter V, Hurd H. Transmission dynamics of malaria in four selected ecological zones of Nigeria in the rainy season. Annals of African Medicine. 2009;**8**(1):1-9. ISSN: 1596-3519

[24] Oyerinde JPO. Essentials of Tropical Medical Parasitology. Akoka: University of Lagos Press; 1999. 435 p. ISBN: 978-017-615-2

[25] WHO. Global Malaria Programme: World Malaria Report. Geneva, Switzerland: World Health Organization; 2010

[26] Federal Ministry of Health (FMH Report). Nigeria Mosquito Control Programme; Federal Ministry of Health, Abuja (Nigerian Strategic Plan); 2009-2013

[27] Okwa OO. Current trends in integrated prevention and control of malaria: A case study of some Nigerian communities. Global Advance Research Journal of Medicine and Medical Sciences. 2013;**2**(4):104-107

[28] Awolola TS, Okwa OO, Hunt RH, Ogunrinade AF. Dynamics of the malaria vector population in coastal Lagos, south-western, Nigeria. Annals of Tropical Medicine and Parasitology. 2002;**96**(1):75-82. DOI: 10.1179/000349802125000538

[29] Awolola TS, Oyewole IO, Koekemoer LL, Coetzee M. Identification of three members within the *Anopheles funestus* group and their role in malaria transmission in two ecological zones in Nigeria. Transactions of the Royal Society for Tropical Medicine and Hygiene. 2005;**99**:525-531

[30] Awolola TS, Bitsindou P, Bagayoko M, Manga L. Malaria Entomological Profile for Nigeria. Geneva, Switzerland: WHO-AFRO Publication; 2007. 50 p

[31] Centre for Disease Control (CDC, 2004): Malaria Report: http://www.cdc.gov/malaria

[32] Oyewole IO, Awolola TS, Ibidapo CA, Okwa OO, Obansa JA. Behavior and population dynamics of the major anopheline vectors in a malaria endemic area in southern Nigeria. Journal of Vector Borne Diseases. 2007;**44**:56-64

[33] Beier JC. Malaria parasite development in mosquitoes. Annual Review of Entomology. 1998;**43**:519-543

[34] Greenwood BM, Da F, Kyle DE. Malaria: Progress, perils and prospects for eradication. Journal of Clinical Investigation. 2008;**118**(4):1266-1276

[35] Okwa OO, Rasheed A, Adeyemi A, Omoyeni M, Oni L, Fayemi A, et al. *Anopheles* species abundance,

composition and vectoral competence in six areas of Lagos, Nigeria. Journal of Cell and Animal Biology. 2007;**1**(2):15-23

[36] Okwa OO, Carter V, Hurd H. Abundances, host preferences and infectivity rates of malaria vectors in Badagry local government area of Lagos, Nigeria. Nigerian Journal of Parasitology. 2006;**27**(1):41-48. ISSN: 1117-4145

[37] Okwa OO, Dennis JO. Malariometric indices of mosquitoes caught outdoors in Iba local council development area (LCDA), Lagos state, Nigeria. Occupational Medicine and Health Affairs. 2015;**3**(3):1-4. DOI: 10.417/2329-6879.1000203

[38] Oyewole IO, Ibidapo CA, Okwa OO, Oduola GO, Adeoye GO, Okoh HI, et al. Species composition and the role of *Anopheles* mosquitoes in malaria transmission along Badagry axis of Lagos lagoon, Nigeria: Libertas Academia. International Journal of Insect Science. 2010;**2**:1-7

[39] Okwa OO, Savage AA. Oviposition and breeding water sites preferences of mosquitoes within Ojo area, Lagos state, Nigeria. Biomedical Journal of Scientific and Technical Research. 2018;**7**(5):1-7. DOI: 10.26717/BJSTR.07.001565

[40] Aju- Ameh OC, Awolola TS, Mwansat GS, Mufuyau HB. Flaws in house design that aid mosquito invasion of human habitat and malaria transmission (a review). Journal of Environmental Science, Toxicology and Food Technology. 2017;**11**:61-69

Chapter 6

Aedes aegypti: The Main Enemy of Public Health in Brazil - Challenges and Perspective for Public Health

Erika M. de Carvalho, Simone S. Valverde and July A.H. Muñoz

Abstract

Mosquitoes (Diptera: Culicidae) are important vectors responsible for transmission of many diseases and parasites. They are causing millions of deaths every year and are considered one of the deadliest animals in the world. The most common arboviruses, such as dengue, chikungunya and Zika, to which the Brazilian population is most exposed and that occur through the bites of the *Aedes aegypti* mosquito, which is the main aim of this study. These infections caused by these three arboviruses are widely distributed on the national territory and have severe consequence to population in some cases. Without effective vaccine and specific treatment, the maintenance and integration of a continuous entomological and epidemiological surveillance are important, besides the methods to control and to prevent these arboviruses in Brazil. This chapter discusses the role of Fiocruz (Oswaldo Cruz Foundation, the most prominent institution of science and technology in health in Latin America) for the development of new methodologies to diagnose and control mosquito-borne diseases through public health policies for the country.

Keywords: *Aedes aegypti*, dengue, Zika, chikungunya, surveillance, prevention

1. Introduction

The mosquitoes' ability of disease transmission is studied since the nineteenth century, although malaria has affected humanity for millennia. Oswaldo Cruz called it "Amazonian's elf," and in the 50th year, a new disease combat method became important worldwide, the medicated salt of Mario Pinotti. Since this, the efforts of the Oswaldo Cruz Foundation (Fiocruz) combated and prevented the diseases transmitted by mosquitoes in Brazil. Among these diseases, we can find malaria, dengue, Zika and chikungunya. Brazilian territory is an endemic area for their transmission, considering the tropical climate and the Brazilian population habits. In the last years, the country was affected by an outbreak caused by chikungunya virus and by the third arbovirus (Zika virus—ZIKV). These viruses were responsible for causing a large number of infections [1, 2].

1.1 *Aedes aegypti*

The first report about *Aedes aegypti* is dated from 1925 by Kirkpatrick, in Egypt [3]. *Aedes aegypti* is a small dark-colored mosquito with white stripes markings. Mosquito is considered domesticated animal as much as other animals, such as the pet dog or cat [3]. These mosquitoes can use natural locations or artificial containers with waters to lay their eggs, thus tree holes, plant axils and common household items that can accumulate rainwater, for example, are potential breeding sites, especially when these locations contain organic material. During their lifetime, the *A. aegypti* females are found around the houses and all day long they are capable of biting humans. Unlike most other mosquitoes, *Aedes* mosquitoes are active and bite only during the daytime, with peak activity during the early morning and in the evening before dusk. They are also capable of biting other animals, but without transmitting diseases to them. Thus, after feeding on human blood, they lay her eggs in the still water. These eggs are laid over a period of several days, and they are resistant to desiccation surviving for long periods of six or more months, until they have contact with water again, and the larvae are released [4, 5].

In America regions, *A. aegypti* is the only epidemiological important species transmitting the dengue virus. This species is originated from Africa where it was domesticated and adapted to the environment created by man, becoming anthropophilic. In the seventeenth century, these mosquitoes started spreading all over the world, to Mediterranean in the eighteenth century, to tropical Asia in the nineteenth century and to Pacific Island in the end of the nineteenth century and beginning of the twentieth century. These adaptive characteristics allowed them to become abundant in many cities and easily carried to other areas by means of transport, which increased their vectorial competence, that is, their ability to become infected by a virus, to replicate it and transmit it. Although *A. aegypti* eradication took place in the Mediterranean in the 1950s and between 1950s and 1960s in most countries of the Americas, there was a reinfestation in most of the areas from which it had been previously eradicated. Nowadays, this vector is considered a cosmotropical species due to the increasing adaptive capacity of the *A. aegypti* [6–10].

In the past, *Aedes albopictus* has its origin in the Asian jungles, but in consequence of an intense tire trade, by sea, this vector came to the Americas in the 1980s, firstly to the USA and then, in Brazil and in others countries of the Central and South America, in Africa, Europe but either in some Pacific Island [6]. *A. albopictus* also lays their eggs in tree holes, but differently of *A. aegypti*, that mosquito has their habits outside the household and bites both animals and humans (anthropophilic and zoophilic diurnal habits). In Asia, *A. albopictus* is responsible for the transmission of epidemic outbreaks of classical and hemorrhagic dengue fever [11].

1.2 Arboviruses: dengue, Zika and chikungunya

Arboviruses (an acronym of ARthropod-BOrne virus) have caused much concern in public health worldwide. Arboviruses have been emerging in different parts of the world due to genetic changes in the virus, alteration of the host and vector population dynamics or because of anthropogenic environmental factors. These viruses' capacity for adaptation is notable, as well as the likelihood of their emergence and establishment in new geographic areas [12]. Here, we highlight three important viruses such as dengue virus (DENV), chikungunya virus (CHIKV), and, lately, Zika virus (ZIKV).

Dengue is a flaviviruses infection transmitted by mosquitoes of *Aedes* genus, mainly *A. aegypti* and *A. albopictus*. The dengue virus (DENV) comprises five distinct serotypes, and this disease is a fast emerging pandemic-prone viral considered the major public health challenge worldwide [4, 13].

The first epidemic of dengue hemorrhagic fever occurred in Manila, Philippines, between 1953 and 1954, followed by Bangkok, Thailand and Malaysia in 1958 and Singapore and Vietnam in 1960. Due to economic growth and consequent increase of post-World War II urbanization, the epidemic of dengue and hemorrhagic dengue spread in the 1970s to other areas of the world, starting in Southeast Asia [10].

In Brazil, since the 1980s, there is an intense virus circulation with epidemic bursts affecting all the regions of the country [14].

The World Health Organization (WHO) estimates 100 million symptomatic cases per year and 2.5 billion people are at risk of infection worldwide. There are no available vaccines and no effective treatment for dengue, which reinforces the need for strategies to prevent virus transmission by the main vector *A. aegypti* (**Figure 1**).

ZIKV is also transmitted by *Aedes aegypti,* and it was first isolated from a rhesus macaque (*Macaca mulatta*) placed as sentinel during a study about yellow fever in the Zika Forest, Uganda, Africa in 1947 [15]. ZIKV had its first documented outbreak only in 2007 in Micronesia. Since then, the transmission area has spread to islands in the Pacific Ocean, especially during a great epidemic in Polynesia in October 2013. In 2015, some cases of humans infected by ZIKV were reported in Brazil, developing into an outbreak that spread throughout South America, the Caribbean islands and Central America. Originally adapted to a zoonotic cycle in Africa, ZIKV evolved into an urban cycle involving a human reservoir and domestic mosquito vectors [16].

Zika virus was first identified in Uganda in 1947. Before 2007, only sporadic human cases were reported from countries in Africa and Asia. In 2007, the first documented Zika virus disease outbreak was reported in the Federated States of Micronesia. In subsequent years, outbreaks of Zika virus disease were identified in countries in Southeast Asia and the Western Pacific. Zika virus was identified for the first time in the Western hemisphere in 2015, when large outbreaks were reported in Brazil. Since then, the virus spread throughout the Americas (**Figure 2**) [17].

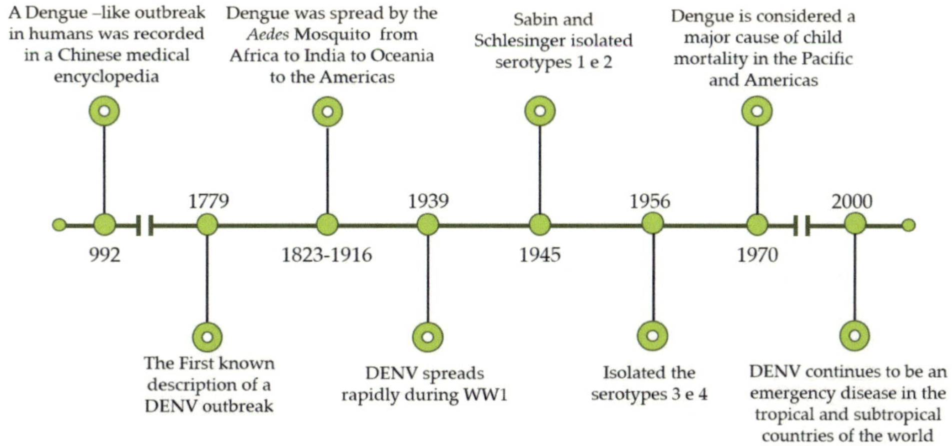

Figure 1.
Chronological spread of DENV (adapted from https://www.centralmosquitocontrol.com/resources/disease-information/dengue).

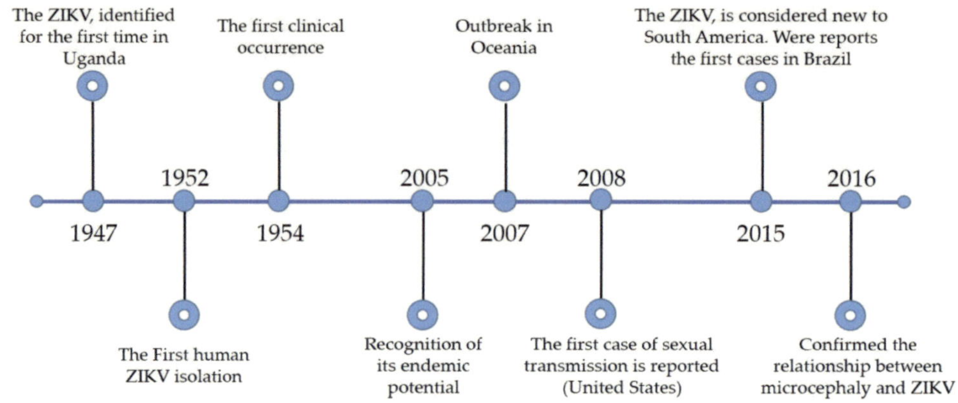

Figure 2.
Chronological spread of ZIKV (adapted from Ref. [18]).

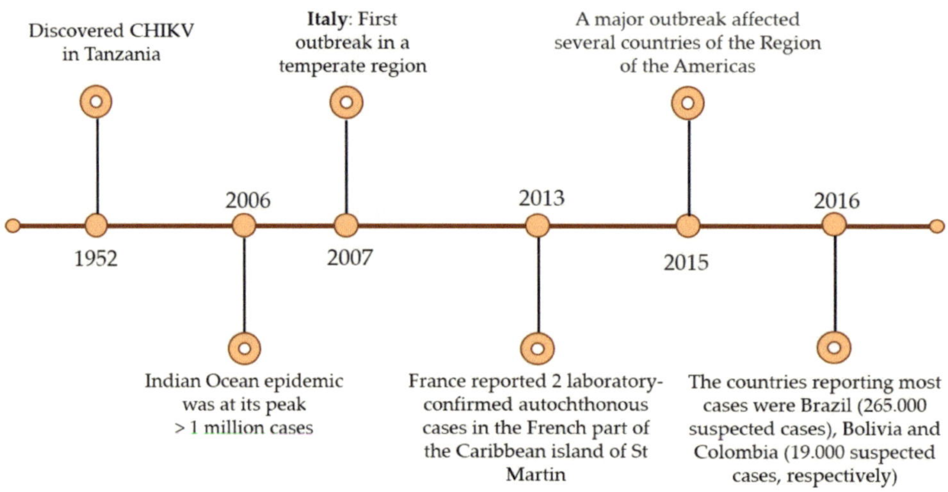

Figure 3.
Chronological spread of CHIKV.

Zika virus caused large outbreaks in previously unexposed populations, and from 2013 onward, outbreaks linked with neurological disorders including Guillain-Barré syndrome and congenital malformations, for reasons that are not yet known. The future transmission of Zika infection is likely to coincide with the global distribution of *Aedes* vectors [19].

A different arbovirus type, an alphavirus, is responsible for causing chikungunya. Differently than the other two diseases, dengue and Zika, chikungunya causes prolonged joint pain and persistent immune response.

Chikungunya is a mosquito-borne viral disease first described during an outbreak in southern Tanzania in 1952. It is an RNA virus that belongs to the alphavirus genus of the family Togaviridae. The name "chikungunya" derives from a word in the Kimakonde language, meaning "to become contorted" and describes the stooped appearance of sufferers with joint pain (arthralgia) (**Figure 3**) [20].

Both *A. aegypti* and *A. albopictus* have been implicated in large outbreaks of chikungunya, whereas *A. aegypti* is confined within the tropics and sub-tropics, *A. albopictus* also occurs in temperate and even cold temperate regions. In recent decades, *A. albopictus* has spread from Asia to become established in areas of Africa, Europe and the Americas [20].

The first report for *A. albopictus* in the Americas occurred in Houston (the United States) in 1985. In Brazil, it was detected for the first time in 1986 in the states of Rio de Janeiro and Minas Gerais [21, 22]. *A. albopictus* was essentially a species wilderness that bred and fed on of the forests and adapted outside houses and inside houses in the various urban and suburban areas of their distribution, according to records made by Gomes and Pessoa [23, 24]. This mosquito species is known as a secondary vector of chikungunya and dengue virus [25].

There is no specific antiviral drug treatment for chikungunya. The treatment is directed primarily at relieving the symptoms, including the joint pain using antipyretics, optimal analgesics and fluids. There is also no commercial chikungunya vaccine.

2. Clinical diagnosis and treatment for dengue, Zika and chikungunya fever

The greatest challenge is the differential clinical diagnosis between dengue, Zika and chikungunya. These three diseases have identical symptomatology and often the patient may present more than one disease at the same time or even having one of these diseases without the manifestation of symptoms. The clinical diagnosis can still occur after some days after the beginning of the infection, but mainly by laboratorial diagnosis [26–28].

Dengue, Zika and chikungunya infection are diagnosed based on clinical, laboratory and epidemiological criteria. It is an important recognition and differentiation of the clinical symptoms and signs to make the correct diagnosis, start proper treatment and prevent the associated complications [26–28].

Dengue is an exanthematic febrile disease, which is often accompanied by nausea, aches (especially frontal headache) and pains and responsible for high rates of morbidity and mortality in countless endemic areas around the world.

In dengue fever, the incubation period lasts for 4–10 days; after that, the disease has three phases: febrile (lasts 2–7 days with no specific signs and symptoms); critical (last 24–48 h) and convalescence. The progression to severe dengue infection (hemorrhagic fever) is variable and difficult to predict [29].

Zika fever and dengue are so similar, characterized by fever, exanthema, headache, conjunctivitis (nonpurulent), myalgia and arthralgia (notably small joints of hands and feet).

Unlike dengue, Zika presents low morbidity, but it is associated by diseases such as congenital microcephaly cases and Guillain-Barré syndrome (a neurological disorder that could lead to paralysis and death), myelitis and meningoencephalitis [30].

Zika fever is very analogous to dengue, symptom manifests in period of 3–12 days and lasts for 4–7 days. It is estimated that in five infected patients, only one develop them [31].

Chikungunya fever symptoms are sudden fever accompanied by headache, polyarthralgia (debilitating) or arthritis and maculopapular rash. The incubation period lasts for 2–12 days. Symptoms usually disappear in less than 2 weeks, but arthralgia may last even years. Severe chikungunya can manifest encephalitis, myocarditis, hepatitis and multiple organ failure that are fatal [32, 33] (**Table 1**).

Diagnosis of dengue, Zika and chikungunya is primarily clinical. In regions of epidemic, dengue is primordial, look for warning symptoms and a complete blood count and transaminases to determinate the phase and severity of the disease. The

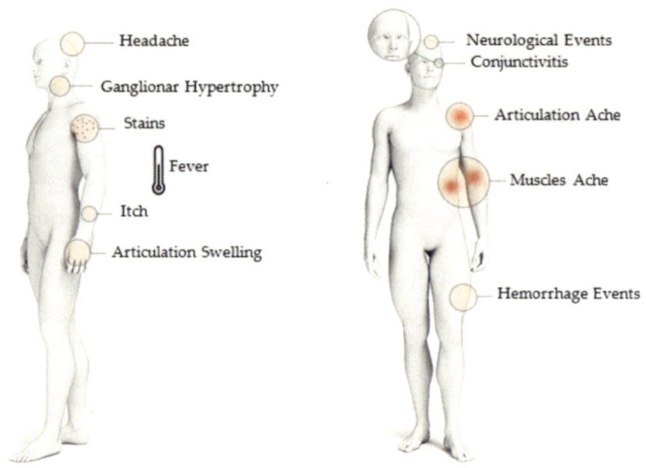

Symptoms*	Arboviruses		
	DENV	CHIKV	ZIKV
Headache	Intense	Moderate	Moderate
Ganglionar hypertrophy	Mild	Moderate	Intense
Cutaneous rash (exantema)	From the 4th day (30–50% cases)	Appear from 2nd and 5th days (50% cases)	Appear from 1st or 2th day (90–100% cases)
Fever	Above 38°C (4–7 days)	Above 38°C (2–3 days)	without febrile and subfebrile 38 (1–2 days of subfebrile)
Itch	Mild	Mild	From moderate to intense
Articulation swelling	Rare	From moderate to intense	Mild
Neurological events	Rare	Rare	More frequently that DENV and CHIKV
Conjunctivitis	Rare	30% cases	50–90% cases
Joint pain	Mild	From moderate to intense	Moderate
Muscles pain	Intense	Intense	Moderate
Hemorrhage events	Moderate	Mild	—

**Adapted from: http://combateaedes.saude.gov.br/pt/sintomas*

Table 1.
The main symptoms of dengue, Zika and chikungunya.

methods for establishing a laboratory diagnosis of these arboviruses are as follows: (1) detection of the virus for example, cell culture or viral RNA real-time detection; (2) antibody detection for example, IgM or IgG detection and (3) antigen/antibody combined detection for example, NS1 and IgM/IgG [27, 28].

These diseases are usually self-limiting with no need for hospitalization except warning signs are observed, especially severe dengue. There are no specific treatments available. Only symptomatic treatment with nonsalicylic analgesics and nonsteroid anti-inflammatories drugs are administrated when dengue infection is discovered. Patients should be advised to drink plenty of fluids to replace fluid lost from sweating, vomiting and others.

DOI: http://dx.doi.org/10.5772/intechopen.79780

3. Epidemiology

The Brazilian regions with the highest incidence and prevalence of these diseases (northeast and southeast region) present a favorable climate for the development of the *Aedes aegypti* (**Figure 4**) and the use of lighter clothes, which cover smaller areas of the body, favoring their exposure.

The number of suspected or confirmed dengue cases reported to the World Health Organization (WHO) is showed in **Figure 5** as well its distribution in the world.

In 2015, the incidence of probable cases of dengue fever (number of cases/100,000 inhabitants), according to Brazilian geographic regions, shows that the

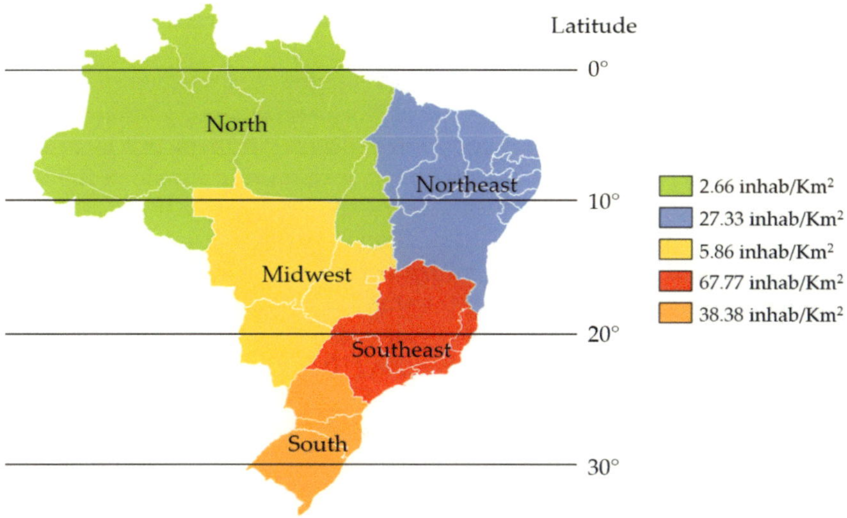

Figure 4.
Brazilian demographic density and latitude at geographic regions.

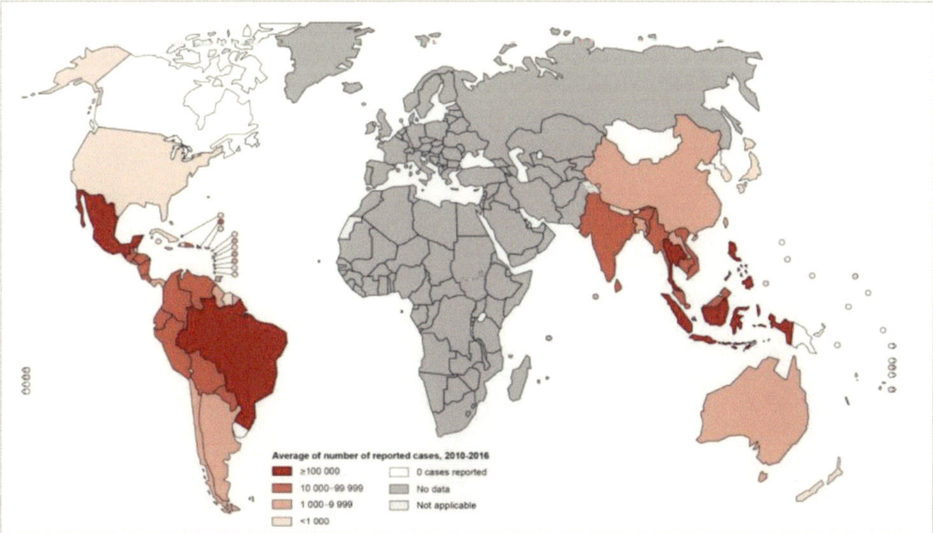

Figure 5.
Average number of suspected or confirmed dengue cases reported to WHO, 2010–2016.

Midwest and Southeast regions had the highest incidence: 1451.9 cases/100,000 inhabitants and 1205.7 cases/100,000 inhabitants, respectively. Among the states, Goiás (2500.6 cases/100,000 inhabitants) and São Paulo (1665.7 cases/100,000 inhabitants) have presented the most incidence numbers [34].

The dengue fever incidence rate was about 733.4 cases/100,000 inhabitants in all Brazilian States at 2016. During this year, the midwest (1322.0/100,000 inhabitants) and the southeast (1001.2/100,000 inhabitants) regions have presented bigger incidence numbers than the other geographic Brazilian regions [35].

In 2017, the midwest region had an incidence of 502.7 cases/100,000 inhabitants and the northeast region had 151.8 cases/100,000 inhabitants, most notably the states of Goiás with 947.3 cases/100.00 inhabitants, Ceará with 453.4/100,000 inhabitants and Tocantins with 331.2/100,000 inhabitants [36].

Figure 6 shows the total number cases of dengue in Brazilian regions during 2015–2017, mainly in the Southeast and Northeast regions, due to their characteristic climate aspects.

In 2015, 38,499 suspected chikungunya fever cases were registered in Brazil (**Figure 6**) which caused an incidence rate of 18.8 cases/100,000 inhabitants. These cases were distributed by 704 cities and 17,971 (46.7%) of them and 14 deaths were confirmed: 05 in Bahia, 02 in Sergipe and 07 in Pernambuco Brazilian states [35].

In 2016, the registered cases number increased significantly to 271,824 and the incidence rate was 133.0 cases/100,000 inhabitants. These cases were distributed in 2829 cities and 151,318 (55.7%) were confirmed. Once again, the northeast region had the highest incidence rate. Among the states were: Rio Grande do Norte (723.1 cases/100,000 inhabitants), Ceará (537.7 cases/100,000 inhabitants), Alagoas (514.8 cases/100,000 inhabitants) and Paraíba (503.0 cases/100,000 inhabitants). At the same year, 196 deaths caused by Chikungunya fever were confirmed [35].

In 2017, the registered cases number had a slight decrease with 185,737, and the incidence rate was 90.1 cases/100,000 inhabitants. However, there are 52,285 cases discarded. During this year, the Northeast region had the highest number of probable chikungunya fever cases (142,131 cases, 76.5%) in relation to the total of the country. Followed by the Southeast (22,984 cases, 12.4%), North (16,570 cases, 8.9%), Midwest (3679 cases, 2.0%) and South (373 cases, 0.2%) [36].

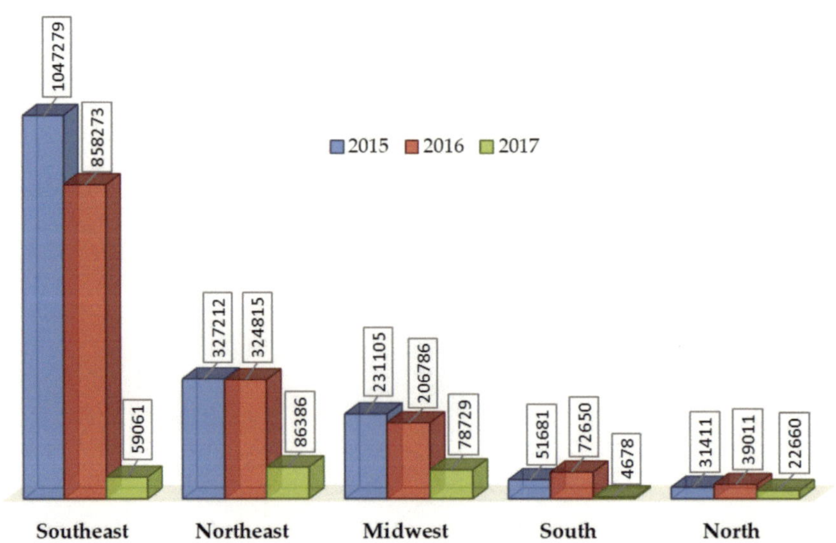

Figure 6.
Total dengue cases within Brazilian regions at the last 3 years.

The analysis of the incidence rate of probable cases of chikungunya fever (number of cases/100,000 inhabitants), according to geographic regions, shows that the Northeast presents the highest incidence rate: 249.7 cases/100,000 inhabitants. Among the Brazilian states, we highlight Ceará (1271.0 cases/100,000 inhabitants), Roraima (795.0 cases/100,000 inhabitants) and Tocantins (207.1 cases/100,000 inhabitants) [36].

The general objective of the Zika surveillance is to describe the epidemiology of the occurrence of microcephaly related to congenital infections in the national territory. Thus, from week 45/2015 until week 06/2016, there were 5280 registered cases of microcephaly occurrence, considering newborns, stillbirths, abortion and fetuses. Considering the year of notification, 60.1% (3174/5280) were recorded in 2015 and 39.9% (2106/5280) in 2016. [37]. Thus 3174 are confirmed, being 508 confirmed and 203 of these cases distributed in 13 Brazilian states, mainly in Northeast region (93.6%). Southeast region presented only five microcephaly notified cases. At least 27 of the confirmed cases evolved to death after birth or during pregnancy. At the end of 2016, the number of reported cases of the microcephaly increased to 10,867. Of these, 3183 (29.3%) remain under investigation and 7684 (70.7%) cases were investigated and classified, being 2366 confirmed, 49 probable and 5269 discarded. According to the geographical distribution, confirmed cases of the 10,867 reported are distributed in 751 Brazilian cities of the 27 Brazilian states, mainly in Northeast region (75.3%). The southeast region showed a large increase in the number of confirmed cases of microcephaly: 74 cases [38].

Due to this epidemiological situation of Zika viruses and its consequences, this disease is considered an Emergency in Public Health of National Importance (ESPIN). From week 45/2015 and until week 52/2017,there were 15,298 cases notified of suspected changes in growth and possibly related to infection with the Zika virus and other infectious etiologies, of which 2869 (18.8%) remained research until 2017, December. Of the total cases, 3071 (20.1%) were confirmed, 339 (2.2%) were classified as likely to be related to infection during pregnancy and 230 (1.5%) as inconclusive. The majority of cases reported is concentrated in the Northeast region of the country (60.6%), followed by the Southeast (23.9%) and Midwest region (7.3%). The five Brazilian states with the greatest number of reported cases are Pernambuco (16.8%), Bahia (16.3%), São Paulo (9.0%), Paraíba (7.3%) and Rio de Janeiro (7.3%) [39].

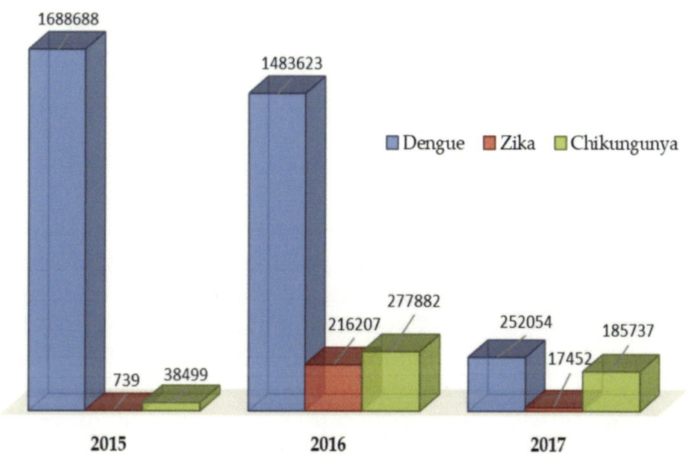

Figure 7.
Cases of dengue, chikungunya and Zika fever in Brazil during 2015, 2016 and 2017.

Nowadays, the 542 microcephaly cases confirmed in Brazil between weeks 1 and 52/2017, 204 (37.6%) received care in childcare. The confirmed children were concentrated in the Southeast (183 cases). Attending in precocious stimulation was performed in 100 of the 542 (18.5%) of confirmed cases, while care in specialized care occurred in 184 of the 542 (33.9%) confirmed cases [39].

Figure 7 shows the behavior of these three diseases in relation to the number of registered cases for the period 2015–2017.

These epidemiology data have demonstrated the incidence rates of the three arboviruses among 2015–2017. In 2016, the incidence of dengue cases has slightly decreased. In 2017, although the numbers of dengue have decreased, the cases of Zika and chikungunya increased, consequently the occurrence of accompany Zika diseases increases during the same period, mainly the microcephaly cases [35–39].

4. Control and prevention

For residents in areas populated by the *Aedes aegypti* species, the most important preventative measure they can take is to remove standing water wherever possible to eliminate breeding sites. This species can breed in as little as one tablespoon of water, so every effort should be made to eliminate standing water in buckets, old tires, gutters, birdbaths, flower pots and more. Additionally, residents should protect themselves indoors with the use of air conditioning and properly maintained window screens and outdoors with the use of mosquito repellents containing DEET (N,N-diethyl-meta-toluamide) and loose fitting clothing [40]. At present, the control of dengue disease is mainly hampered by the absence of antivirals or a vaccine, which results in an estimated half worldwide population at risk of infection.

Currently, antiviral treatment against dengue is available, and the development of an effective anti-dengue vaccine would represent a cornerstone in public health. An important aspect of dengue is that an effective immunity can be potentially impaired during heterologous infections (refers to the immunity that can develop to one pathogen after a host has had exposure to nonidentical pathogens), which may lead to severe manifestations of dengue and represents a great burden in the development of a vaccine against this pathogen.

Due to the absence of an effective vaccine for these arboviruses, the control is still accomplished through the prevention and elimination of potential mosquito-breeding habitats. Thus, the use of chemical insecticides is yet the main vector control component. Alternative products, with potential to be used in the control of *A. aegypti*, including the biolarvicide Bti (*Bacillus thuringiensis var. israelensis*) and some insect growth regulators are also being used recently [41].

4.1 Vaccination

It is widely recognized that passive vaccination is the most appropriate preventive and therapeutic option but till now no vaccine is available for Zika and chikungunya although some initiative to the development of a vaccine have been tested. Several vaccine approaches have been used such as inactivated viral vaccines, live-attenuated viruses, recombinant subunit vaccines, DNA vaccination and others. In Brazil, a live-attenuated viruses vaccine developed by Sanofi Pasteur laboratory has been available since 2016. It is sold in private clinics and is part of vaccination pilot public programs in Paraná state. The product requires three applications with an interval of 6 months between them. In the early studies, the efficacy in the population above 9 years old is approximately 66% against the four serotypes of dengue virus. In addition, it reduces severe cases—those that lead to death, such as hemorrhagic dengue—by 93% and hospitalization rates by 80%.

Pending vaccine development, the measures recommended to prevent against mosquito bites and vector control consist of individual protection or action. Mosquito control is the best available method for preventing arboviruses infection. Breeding sites must be removed, destroyed, cleaned and treated with insecticides.

4.2 Repellents and larvicides

About the intervention against mosquitoes, mainly *Aedes aegypti*, the use of new repellents and insecticides agents are investigated. Due to the development of resistance, biological magnification of toxic substances through the food chain, and others adverse effects on the environment and human health caused by the synthetic insecticides, eco-friendly agents control of mosquitoes vectors have a great importance to avoid dengue, Zika and chikungunya and others diseases transmitted by *A. aegypti*. By this way, so many natural products as plant extracts and essential oils have been evaluated against larval and pupal stages of *A. aegypti* as nanoparticles containing plant extracts and the essential oils from *Zingiber officinale, Curcuma longa, Ocimum basilicum,* and *Mentha piperita* which variety of types and levels of their actives constituents could be responsible for their potential to combat mosquitoes and have been shown to be promising and low-cost mosquitoes control strategies [42–45].

Other intervention, could be done such as using repellents with DEET, wear cloth which minimizes skin exposure to the day-biting vectors, stay in places with air conditioning, use domestic insecticides in aerosol form or in vaporizers within the home.

The conventional methods such as insecticides and larval biological used until now revealed that control have proven ineffective at halting disease spreading [46, 47]. A successful system controlling a broad spectrum of approaches should be mutually compatible and encompass including the development of novel insecticides, transgenic disease-resistant mosquitoes, the release of sterile insects to suppress vector populations and equipment for preventing mosquito bites is to be developed [48].

In Brazil, some new approaches to control mosquito have shown considerable promise in latest years are the biolarvicide Bti, the genetic control of *A. aegypti* mosquitoes and the development of mosquitoes that are resistant to arbovirus infection [47].

Brazil was among the pioneers in adopting Bti to control mosquitoes and black flies. Developed by research groups in Brazilian institutions, this bacterial larvicide is highly toxic at very low doses to target organisms (mosquito and black flies larvae) and safe to other nontarget organisms. Larvicidal activity is due to large amounts of crystal proteins produced during sporulation and transformed into toxins under specific conditions after ingestion by larvae. The structure of the proteins made by the bacterium strain and the presence of proteolytic enzymes and receptor in the host larvae midgut determined the selectivity observed. Brazilian product showed some advantages such as reduction in the number of applications, formulation with high storage stability, no environmental impact and high persistence in the environment and especially efficient in tropical climates [49].

4.3 Biological control of mosquitoes

One way to control mosquitoes is the genetic control strategy known as release of insects carrying dominant lethal genes (RIDL) which is an advancement of the environmentally benign sterile insect technique (SIT). The RIDL involves the insertion of a lethal gene into male mosquitoes that prevents them from being able to reproduce successfully. The insects are considered sterile because the vast majority dies before maturing. These genetically modified males will seek out females to mate with and the ensuing progeny will contain the lethal gene [50–52]. If an appropriate number of mosquitoes are released, the females will be more likely to find a modified male, and a substantial drop in population can be achieved in a remarkably short period. To control populations with this technique as "zones" of release should be established to ensure sufficient area coverage. The preliminary results in Brazil showed that successful approach achieved a 95% reduction in local mosquito populations [53].

Another alternative approach to *A. aegypti* control is the use of mosquitoes with the *Wolbachia pipientis* an endosymbiotic bacterium to prevent arboviruses replicating within the mosquito. The bacteria can hinder the fertility of their hosts and influence the sex of offspring. Besides, it can block viruses from reproducing in infected fruit flies and mosquitoes [50, 52, 53]. Mosquito control is an effective measure to prevent a dengue outbreak [54].

FIOCRUZ's initiative to produce, create and release adult mosquitoes infected by bacterium of *Wolbachia* genus in several districts of the city of Rio de Janeiro has been shown to be very effective in controlling the diseases transmitted by *Aedes aegypti*.

Other mosquitoes genetically modified (Moscamed™, created in 2005) are produced in large scale and released in different cities of Bahia states, reducing the mosquito population in 95% during 6 months. These strategies are being expanded throughout the Brazilian territory to combat *Aedes aegypti* [55, 56].

4.4 Control of mosquitoes by the Brazilian government

- Monthly/bimonthly inspection of households/population orientation by health agents;

- Application of larvicides in the houses (more than 300,000 nonmilitary health agents +220,000 soldiers fighting against potential mosquitoes breeding sites);

- Smoke dispersion containing neurotoxic agent to adult mosquitoes at epidemic locals;

- Biological control through the use of a bacterium naturally found in the environment, *Wolbachia*, which when present in *Aedes*, is able to prevent the transmission of the disease by the mosquitoes, and this characteristic is passed through on to their larvae.

5. The role of Fiocruz

In Brazil, dengue has a seasonal pattern, with a higher incidence of cases in the first 5 months of the year, a warmer and wetter period, typical of tropical climates. In the second half of the twentieth century, from 1986, dengue became epidemiologically important, when the epidemic broke out in the State of Rio de Janeiro and the circulation of serotype 1, which soon reached the Northeast Region. Thus, dengue became endemic in Brazil, interspersed with epidemics, usually associated with the introduction of new serotypes, in areas previously indene [14, 55–58].

The Oswaldo Cruz Foundation (Fiocruz), under the Ministry of Health have a mission to produce, disseminate and share knowledge and technologies aimed at the strengthening and consolidation of the Unified Health System (SUS) and contribute to the promotion of health and quality of life of the population [59].

Since 2003, in order to promote dengue control actions, Fiocruz has established the Fiocruz Dengue Network, through the allocation of resources to the Program for Development and Technological Innovation in Public Health in the field of research.

With the epidemiological cycles of the disease continuing, repeating itself and spreading throughout the country, more than 30,000 cases of dengue fever were reported in the city of Rio de Janeiro in 2008. Due to this epidemic, Fiocruz was called to assist the state and municipality in actions to combat the disease.

Thus, from 2009, Fiocruz redirected an integral focus to the issue with coverage in these three areas, without excluding the research. The Network Health Care of Integrated Actions for Health Care in Dengue Control originated from 2015 onwards and began to include in its scope the issues related to two emerging viruses in Brazil: chikungunya and Zika.

Aiming to reduce or even block the transmission of Zika, dengue and chikungunya Fiocruz has set up a factory for the large-scale release of *Aedes aegypti Wolbachia* bacterium in Rio de Janeiro. The plant has the capacity to produce 10 million eggs of the mosquito per week.

The initiative, officially called "Eliminating Dengue: Brazil Challenge," began in 2016 as a pilot project focused on the city of Niterói and the Tubiacanga neighborhood of Rio. According to the project's schedule, it will expand to North and South zones of Rio de Janeiro. The release of mosquitoes will be finalized by the end of 2018, at which time the project's coverage will have increased to a total area occupied by approximately 2.5 million people.

The Oswaldo Cruz Foundation (Fiocruz) developed a new test that will help drive public policies to fight the health emergency caused by the three infection diseases. The kit uses molecular diagnostics to detect and differentiate simultaneous RNA of the three viruses through real-time PCR technology, and the result is released on the same day. The kit can be used for laboratory diagnosis of all three viruses, two of them or each separately. The test allows diagnosis in the critical phase of the disease, at the beginning of clinical symptoms and an accurate laboratory diagnosis is essential. The opportunity or earlier diagnosis can also aid for epidemiological surveillance and prevention of new cases.

Fiocruz maintains investment in research, development and innovation because this is the only way to seek and find answers to the challenges due to triple Zika-dengue-chikungunya epidemic. Therefore, the goal is to search for cooperation with other institutions in Brazil and internationally to build projects that could offer new possibilities to generate knowledge and developing technologies.

6. Conclusion

Aedes aegypti is still a worldwide threat, since more than half of the world's population live in areas where these mosquitoes species are present. However, many efforts have been undertaken to combat and to control these mosquitoes and the diseases transmitted by them, such as vaccination, repellents and larvicides and the biological control of mosquitoes. Brazil has been continuously developing public policies to health education, alerting the population on the risks which can be avoided, with the purpose of decreasing the dengue, Zika and chikungunya diseases. The Brazilian government plays a role in continuing investment in research, development and innovation to find new ways with national and international cooperation to combat *Aedes aegypti*.

Acknowledgements

The authors are grateful to Farmanguinhos and Fiocruz for their financial support.

Conflict of interest

The authors confirm that this chapter content has no conflict of interest.

Abbreviations

CDC	Centers for Disease Control and Prevention
CHIKV	Chikungunya virus
DENV	Dengue virus
DEET	N,N-diethyl-meta-toluamide
ESPIN	Emergency in Public Health of National Importance
FIOCRUZ	Oswaldo Cruz Foundation (A Brazilian Government Research Institute)
IgG	Immunoglobulin G
IgM	Immunoglobulin M
RIDL	release of insects carrying dominant lethal genes
SIT	sterile insect technique
SUS	Unified Health System
WHO	World Health Organization
ZIKV	Zika virus

Author details

Erika M. de Carvalho*, Simone S. Valverde and July A.H. Muñoz
Medicines and Drugs Technology Institute (Farmanguinhos), Oswaldo Cruz Foundation, Rio de Janeiro, RJ, Brazil

*Address all correspondence to: erikamc.far@gmail.com

References

[1] Patterson J, Sammon M, Dengue GM. Zika and chikungunya: Emerging arboviruses in the new world. Western Journal of Emergency Medicine. 2016; **17**(6):671-679. DOI: 10.5811/westjem.2016.9.30904

[2] Cavalcanti LPG, Freitas ARR, Brasil P, Da Cunha RV. Surveillance of deaths caused by arboviruses in Brazil: From dengue to chikungunya. Memórias do Instituto Oswaldo Cruz. 2017;**112**(8): 583-585. DOI: 10.1590/0074-027601 60537

[3] Shoukry NM, Elwan NA, Morsy TA. *Aedes aegypti* (Linnaeus) re-emerging in southern Egypt. Journal of the Egyptian Society of Parasitology. 2012;**42**(1): 41-50. DOI: 10.12816/0006293

[4] World Health Organization (WHO). What is dengue? [Internet] 2017. Available from: http://www.who.int/dengue control/disease/en/ [Accessed: 2017-12-12]

[5] Centers for Disease Control and Prevention (CDC). Dengue and the *Aedes aegypti* mosquito. [Internet]. 2015. Available from: https://www.cdc.gov/dengue/resources/factSheets/factsheet_dengue-what-you-need-to-know.pdf [Accessed: 2017-12-12]

[6] Rodhain F, Rosen L. Mosquito vectors and dengue virus-vector relations ships. In: Gubler DJ, Kuno G, editors. Dengue and Dengue Hemorragic Fever. New York: CAB International; 1997. pp. 45-60

[7] Silva AM, Dittus WPJ, Amerasinghe PH, Amerasinghe FP. Serologic evidence for an epizootic dengue virus infecting toque macaques (*Macaca Sinica*) at Polonnaruwa, Sri Lanka. The American Journal of Tropical Medicine and Hygiene. 1999;**60**(2):300-306. DOI: 10.1002/ajp.10105

[8] Dye C. The analysis of parasite transmission by bloodsuccking insects. Annual Review of Entomology. 1992;**37**: 1-19. DOI: 10.1146/annurev.en.37. 010192.000245

[9] Scott WT, Clark GG, Lorenz LH, Amerasinghe PH, Reiter P, Edman J. Detection of multiple blood feeding in *Aedes aegypti* (*Diptera: culicidae*) during a single gonotrophic cycle using a histologique technique. Journal of Medical Entomology. 1993;**30**(1):94-99. DOI: 10.1093/jmedent/30.1.94

[10] Gubler DJ. Epidemic dengue/ dengue hemorrhagic fever as a public health, social and economic problem in the 21st century. Trends in Microbiology. 2002;**10**(2):100-103. DOI: 10.1016/S0966-842X(01)02288-0

[11] Teixeira MG, Barreto ML, Guerra A. Epidemiologia e medidas de prevenção do Degue. Informe Epidemiológico do SUS. 1999;**8**:5-33

[12] Donalisio MR, Freitas ARR, Zuben V APB. Arboviruses emerging in Brazil: Challenges for clinic and implications for public health. Revista de Saúde Pública. 2017;**51**:30-36. DOI: 10.1590/ S1518-8787.2017051006889

[13] Mustafa MS, Rasotgi V, Jain S, Gupta V. Discovery of fifth serotype of dengue virus (DENV-5): A new public health dilemma in dengue control. Medical Journal Armed Forces India. 2015;**71**(1):67-70. DOI: 10.1016/j. mjafi.2014.09.011

[14] Braga IA, Valle D. *Aedes aegypti*: Histórico do controle no Brasil. Epidemiologia e Serviços de Saúde. 2007;**16**(2):113-118. DOI: 10.5123/ S1679-49742007000200006

[15] Dick GW, Kitchen SF, Haddow AJ. Zika virus. I. Isolations and serological

specificity. Transactions of the Royal Society of Tropical Medicine and Hygiene. 1952;**46**:509-520. DOI: 10.1016/0035-9203(52)90042-4

[16] Epelboin Y, Talaga S, Epelboin L, Dusfour I. Zika virus: An updated review of competent or naturally infected mosquitoes. PLoS Neglected Tropical Diseases. 2017; **11**(11):1-22. DOI: 10.1371/journal.pntd.0005933

[17] Tai-Ho Chen J, Staples E, Fischer M. Infectious diseases related to travel. [Internet]. Available from: https://wwwnc.cdc.gov/travel/yellowbook/2018/infectious-diseases-related-to-travel/zika [Accessed: 2017-12-01]

[18] Dos Santos FB, Nunes PCG, De Sequeira PC, Machado LN, Lima MA, Gava RP. Zika. In: Dengue, Zika E Chikungunya: Diagnóstico, tratamento e prevenção. Organização Luiz José de Souza 1 ed. Rio de Janeiro: Rubio; 2016. 204 p

[19] Kindhauser MK, Allen T, Frank V, Santhanaa RS, Dyea C. Zika: The origin and spread of a mosquito-borne virus. Bulletin of the World Health Organization. 2016;**94**:675-686. DOI: 10.2471/BLT.16.171082

[20] World Health Organization (WHO). Chikungunya [Internet]. Available from: http://www.who.int/mediacentre/factsheeeets/fs327/en/ [Accessed: 2017-11-10]

[21] Forattini OP. Identificação de Aedes (Stegomyia) albopictus no Brasil. Revista de Saúde Pública. 1986;**20**(3): 244-245. DOI: 10.1590/S0034-89101986000300009

[22] Carvalho RG, De Oliveira, RL, Braga IA. Updating the geographical distribution and frequency of *Aedes albopictus* in Brazil with remarks regarding its range in the Americas. Memórias do Instituto Oswaldo Cruz. 2014;**109**(6):787-796. DOI: 10.1590/0074-0276140304

[23] Gomes AC, Souza JMP, Bergamaschi DP, Santos JLF, Andrade VR, Leite OF, et al. Atividade antropofílica de *Aedes aegypti* e Aedes albopictus em área sob controle e vigilância. Revista da Sociedade Brasileira de Medicina Tropical. 2005;**39**(2):206-210. DOI: 0.1590/S0034-86822005000200010

[24] Pessoa VEM, Silveira DA, Cavalcante ILR, Florindo MIG. Aedes albopictus no Brasil: Aspectos ecológicos e riscos de transmissão da dengue. Entomotropica. 2013;**28**(2):75-86

[25] Di Luca M, Severini F, Toma L, Boccolini D, Romi R, Remoli ME. Experimental studies of susceptibility of Italian *Aedes albopictus* to Zika virus. Euro Surveillance. 2016;**21**:30223. DOI: 10.2807/1560-7917.ES.2016.21.18.30223

[26] Beltrán-Silva SL, Chacón-Hernández SS, Moreno-Palacios E, Pereyra-Molina JA. Clinical and diferencial diagnosis: Dengue, chikungunya and zika. Revista Médica del Hospital General de México. 2016; **81**(3):146-153. DOI: 10.1016/j.hgmx.2016.09.011

[27] Tilak R, Ray SCS, Tilak VW, Mukherij S. Dengue, chikungunya and the missing entity—Zika fever: A new emerging threat. Medical Journal Armed Forces India. 2016;**72**:157-163. DOI: 10.106/j.mjafi.2016.02.017

[28] Moulin E, Selby K, Cherpillod P, Kaiser I, Boillat-Blanco N. Simultaneous outbreaks of dengue, chikungunya and zika virus infections: Diagnosis challenge in a returning traveler with nonspecific febrile illness. New Microbes and New infections. 2016;**11**: 6-7. DOI: 10.106/j.nnmi.2016.02.003

[29] Tang KF, Ooi EE. Diagnosis of dengue: An update. Expert Review of

Anti-Infective Therapy. 2012;**10**(8): 895-907. DOI: 10.1586/eri.12.76

[30] WHO. Zika virus and complications: Questions and answers. [Internet]. 2017. Available from: http:// www.who.int/features/qa/zika/en/ [Accessed: 2018-15-01]

[31] Rather IA, Kumar S, Bajpaj VK, Lim J, Park Y-H. Prevention and control strategies to counter zika epidemic. Frontiers in Microbiology. 2017;**8**: 305-413. DOI: 10.3389/fmicb.2017. 00305

[32] Galán-Huerta KA, Rivas-Estilla AM, Férnadez-Sala I, Farfan-Ale JA, Ramos-Jimenéz J. Chikungunya vírus: A general overview. Medicina Universitaria. 2015; **17**(68):175-183. DOI: 10.106/j. rmu.2015.06.001

[33] Caglioti C, Lalle E, Castilletti CF, Capobianchi MR, Bordi L. Chikungunya virus infection: An overview. The New Microbiologica. 2013;**36**:211-227

[34] Brasil, Ministério da Saúde (MS). Monitoramento dos casos de dengue, febre de chikungunya e febre pelo vírus Zika até a Semana Epidemiológica 52, 2015. Boletin epidemiológico. 2016; **47**(3):1-10. ISSN: 2358-9450

[35] Brasil, Ministério da Saúde (MS). Monitoramento dos casos de dengue, febre de chikungunya e febre pelo vírus Zika até a Semana Epidemiológica 52, 2016. Boletin epidemiológico. 2017; **48**(3):1-11. ISSN 2358-9450

[36] Brasil, Ministério da Saúde (MS). Monitoramento dos casos de dengue, febre de chikungunya e febre pelo vírus Zika até a Semana Epidemiológica 52, 2017. Boletin epidemiológico. 2018; **49**(2):1-13. ISSN 2358-9450

[37] Brasil, Ministério da Saúde (MS). Informe Epidemiológico N°13. Monitoramento dos casos de microcefalia no Brasil. [Internet]. 2017. Available from: http://portalarquivos2. saude.gov.br/images/pdf/2016/fevere iro/17/coes-microcefalia-inf-epi-13-se 06-2016.pdf [Accessed: 2018-15-03]

[38] Brasil, Ministério da Saúde (MS). Informe Epidemiológico N°57. Monitoramento dos casos de microcefalia no Brasil. [Internet]. 2017. Available from: http://combateaedes.sa ude.gov.br/images/pdf/Informe-Epide miologico-n57-SE-52_2016-09jan2017. pdf [Accessed: 2018-15-03]

[39] Brasil, Ministério da Saúde (MS). Monitoramento integrado de alterações no crescimento e desenvolvimento relacionadas à infecção pelo vírus Zika e outras etiologias infecciosas, até a Semana Epidemiológica 52 de 2017. Boletin epidemiológico. 2018;**49**(6): 1-10. ISSN 2358-9450

[40] Central Life Sciences. Dengue fever: What you need to know. [Internet]. Available from: https://www.centra lmosquitocontrol.com/resources/disea se-information/dengue [Accessed: 2017-11-10]

[41] Braga IA, Valle D. *Aedes aegypti*: Inseticidas, mecanismos de ação e resistência. Epidemiologia e Serviços de Saúde. 2007;**16**(4):279-293. DOI: 10.5123/S1679-49742007000400006

[42] Govindarajan M, Rajeswary M, Mutukumaran U, Hoti SL, Khater HF, Benelli G. Single-step biosynthesis and characterization of silver nanoparticles using *Zornia dphylla* leaves: A pontent eco-friendly tool against malaria and arbovirus vectors. Journal of Photochemistry and Photobiology. B. 2016;**161**:482-489. DOI: 10.1016/j. jphotobiol.2016.06.016

[43] Govindarajan M, Khater HF, Panneerslvan C, Benelli G. One-pot fabrication of silver nanocrystals using *Nicandra physalodes:* A novel route for mosquito vector control with moderate toxicity on non-target water bugs.

Research in Veterinary Science. 2016; **107**:95-101. DOI: 10.1016/j.rvsc.2016.05.017

[44] Roni M, Murugan K, Panneerselvam C, Subramaniam J, Nicoletti M, Madhiyazhagan P, et al. Characterization and biotoxicity of *Hypnea musciformis*-synthesized silver nanoparticles as potential eco-friendly control tool against *Aedes aegypti* and *Plutella xylostella*. Ecotoxicology and Environmental Safety. 2015;**121**:31-38. DOI: 10.1016/j.ecoenv.2015.07.005

[45] Khater HF. Bioactivity of essential oils as green. In: Govil JN, Bhattacharya S, editors. Recent Progress in Medicinal Plants, Vol. 37. Essential Oils II. 2013. pp. 153-220

[46] Maciel-de-Freitas R, Peres RC, Alves F, Brandolini MB. Mosquito traps designed to capture *Aedes aegypti* (Diptera: Culicidae) females: Preliminary comparison of Adultrap, MosquiTRAP and backpack aspirator efficiency in a dengue-endemic area of Brazil. Memórias do Instituto Oswaldo Cruz. 2008;**103**:602-605. DOI: 10.1590/S0074-02762008000600016

[47] Faucon F, Dusfour I, Gaude T, Navratil V, Boyer F, Chandre F, et al. Identifying genomic changes associated with insecticide resistance in the dengue mosquito *Aedes aegypti* by deep targeted sequencing. Genome Research. 2015; **25**(9):1347-1359. DOI: 10.1101/gr.189225.115

[48] Khater HF. Ecosmart biorational insecticides: Alternative insect control strategies. In: Perveen F, editor. Insecticides—Advances in Integrated Pest Management. InTech; 2012. DOI: 10.5772/27852. Available from: https://www.intechopen.com/books/insecticides-advances-in-integrated-pest-management/ecosmart-biorational-insecticides-alternative-insect-control-strategies

[49] Sanches EG, da Silva ACB, Campos FMA, Pinheiro RA, de Jesus FJ. Composição bioinseticida à base de *Bacillus thuringiensis* var israelensis e o respectivo processo de preparação. Patente: PI0003314-6. Concedida em 24 de maio de 2000

[50] Yakob L, Walker T. Zika virus outbreak in the Americas: The need for novel mosquito control methods. The Lancet Global Health. 2016;**4**(3): e148-e149. DOI: 10.1016/S2214-109X(16)00048-6

[51] Alphey L. Genetic control of mosquitoes. Annual Review of Entomology. 2014;**59**(1):205-224. DOI: 10.1146/annurev-ento-011613-162002

[52] McGraw EA, O'Neill SL. Beyond insecticides: New thinking on an ancient problem. Microbiology. 2013;**11**:181-193. DOI: 10.1038/nrmicro2968

[53] Dutra HLC, Rocha MN, Stehling FB, Mansur SB, Caragata, EP, Moreira L. Wolbachia blocks currently circulating zika virus isolates in Brazilian *Aedes aegypti* mosquitoes. Cell Host & Microbe. 2016;**19**(6):771-774. DOI: 10.1016/j.chom.2016.04.021

[54] Pang T, Mak TK, Gubler DJ. Prevention and control of dengue—The light at the end of the tunnel. The Lancet Infectious Diseases. 2017;**17**:79-87

[55] Ministry of Health. Secretariat of Social Communication—International Area Presidency of the Federative Republic of Brazil. 2016

[56] Carvalho DO, McKemey AR, Garziera L, Lacroix R, Donnelly CA, Alphey L, et al. Suppression of a field population of *Aedes aegypti* in Brazil by sustained release of transgenic male mosquitoes. PLoS Neglected Tropical Diseases. 2015;**9**:e0003864. DOI: 10.1371/journal.pntd.0003864

[57] Schatzmayr HG. Dengue situation by year 2000. Memórias do Instituto Oswaldo Cruz. 2000;**95**:179-181. DOI: 10.1590/S0074-02762000000700030

[58] Silva JB Jr, Siqueira JB Jr, Coelho GE, Vilarinhos PT, Pimenta FG Jr. Dengue in Brazil: Current situation and control activities. Epidemiological Bulletin. 2002;**23**(1):3-6

[59] FIOCRUZ The Foundation [Internet]. Available from: https://portal.fiocruz.br/en/content/foundation [Accessed: 2017-11-10]

Chapter 7

New Cost-Benefit of Brazilian Technology for Vector Surveillance Using Trapping System

Alvaro E. Eiras, Marcelo C. Resende, José L. Acebal and Kelly S. Paixão

Abstract

The recent introduction of chikungunya and Zika virus and their subsequent dispersion in the Americas have encouraged the use of novel technologies for adult *Aedes* surveillance to improve vector control. In Brazil, two platforms for surveillance of eggs and gravid *Aedes aegypti* have been developed. First, it consists of using data of sampling of eggs in ovitraps associated with GIS technologies to monitor *Aedes* spp. populations. Although effective, it is not realistic to use in a large-scale epidemic scenario as it requires a large amount of human resources for field and laboratory activities. Second, it consists of trapping female *Ae. aegypti* citywide at fine spatial and temporal scales for vector surveillance (MI-*Aedes*) to detect high *Aedes* infestation areas using a GIS environment and the identification of arbovirus-infected trapped mosquitoes by RT-PCR (MI-Virus platforms). Such integration of continuous vector surveillance and targeting vector control in hotspot areas is cost-effective (less than US$ 1.00/person/year), and it has been shown to reduce mosquito population and prevent dengue transmission. The main advantage of the MI-*Aedes* platform over traditional mosquito surveillance is the integration of continuous vector monitoring coupled with an information technology platform for near real-time data collection, analysis, and decision-making. The technologies also provide data to model the role of climate on the vector population dynamics.

Keywords: surveillance, vector control, novel technologies, adult trap, MI-*Aedes*, MI-Virus

1. Introduction

The public health impact of arthropod-borne viruses (arboviruses) has increased dramatically over the last 50 years with diseases such dengue and chikungunya spreading to new geographic locations and increasing in incidence [1]. Most of the known arboviruses were initially isolated in tropical areas such as Africa, South America, and some Asian countries [2]. In fact, many of the diseases transmitted by arthropods encountered today not only existed but were widespread in their distribution before written records began and are among the major causes of illness and death in many countries. In recent years, and despite efforts to control vectors, the prevalence of viral infections transmitted by arthropods worldwide has increased. However, changes in viral genetics, host, and vector population as well as the global climate facilitated, among other factors, the expansion and spread of arboviruses in the world. The expansion of global human population, migratory movements of people and animals, and rapid disordered urbanization led to a closer contact between man and animal reservoirs, thereby increasing exposure to infection with arboviruses [2].

Various arboviruses including the important public health concern dengue virus (DENV) [3], yellow fever virus [4], chikungunya virus (CHIKV) [5], and Zika virus (ZIKV) [6] have *Aedes aegypti* (**Figure 1**) and *Aedes albopictus* as vectors. The most prevalent human arboviral infection is caused by DENV that accounts for approximately 100 million annual infections worldwide with almost half of the world's population at risk of infection [7, 8]. Since CHIKV was firstly detected in the Americas in December 2013, it has caused more than 1.7 million of confirmed or suspected cases. At least 48 countries and territories of the Americas confirmed the autochthonous circulation of ZIKV [9].

Historically, surveillance of vectors that transmit arboviruses was focused on immature stages (eggs, larvae, and pupae) with little emphasis given to the adult mosquito. The oviposition trap (ovitrap) developed in the 1960s [10] is still being used to detect *Aedes* spp., especially when vector population is low (**Figure 2a**). However, surveillance of adult female population is necessary to evaluate the impact of vector control interventions, to detect arboviruses, and to look for insecticide resistance alleles. Interventions that also require surveillance of adult mosquito population include evaluations on the efficacy of insecticide-treated materials, the release of sterile or genetically modified insects, and the dispersion of spatial repellents.

In light of the requirements listed above, various traps have been developed to monitor the populations of *Aedes* spp. and other arthropods by sampling eggs and host-seeking or gravid females. Traps devised to catch adult *Ae. aegypti* are divided into two major classes: active and passive. Passive traps are low cost and capture gravid *Ae. aegypti* without electricity using funnels, sticky cards, or insecticides. In these traps, water or an infusion of hay is used to attract the insects. Examples of sticky traps for adult vectors are MosquiTRAP, Gravid *Aedes* Trap (GAT), and Autocidal Gravid Ovitrap (CDC-AGO) (**Figure 2b–d**) [11]. The catch rates of passive traps depend on factors such as size, color, and type of attractant, among others. In contrast, active traps use an electrical device—for instance, a battery-operated fan that sucks the insects into the trap. BG-Sentinel (**Figure 2e**) is an example of active trap used to capture adult mosquitoes.

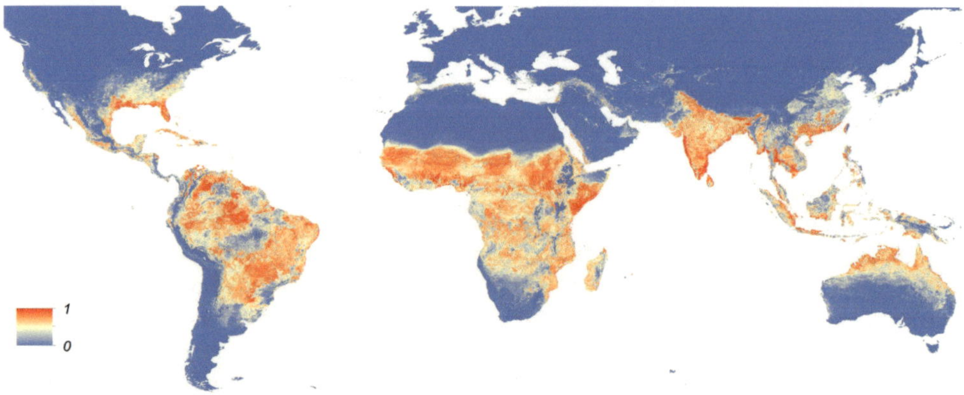

Figure 1.
Global map of forecasted probability of occurrence of Aedes aegypti at a spatial resolution of 5 × 5 km (Kraemer et al. [1], https://doi.org/10.7554/eLife.08347.004).

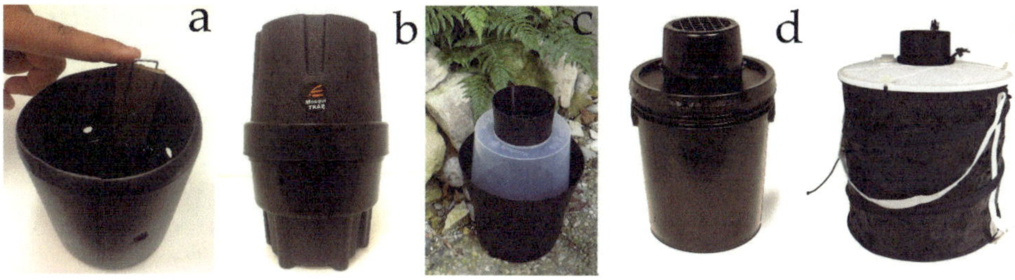

Figure 2.
Passive mosquito traps used for surveillance: (a) ovitrap, (b) MosquiTRAP, (c) Aedes Gravid Traps (GAT), (d) Autocidal Gravid Ovitrap (CDC-AGO), and (e) the active trap BG-Sentinel.

Health authorities are increasingly employing new technologies in order to achieve integrated *Aedes* management. In this context, predictive mathematical modeling has the potential to help authorities to act preemptively by rapidly preparing vector alerts and mobilizing the resources needed for an integrated vector management whenever an imminent surge of mosquitoes and, therefore, a higher risk of infection with arboviruses are likely to take place. Also, by assessing the data collected by surveillance traps for adult mosquitoes using spatial statistics, it is possible to present data correlating the infestation index with other variables such as the vector control method used, epidemiological data, virus-infected mosquito data, and climatic data, among others [12]. The automated presentation of the results obtained directly from the field allows the integrated analysis of entomological data with geographic information system (GIS), thereby enabling the deliverance of immediate vector control responses to the precise localities presenting the highest levels of mosquito infestation.

Climate is an important factor in the geographic and temporal distribution of arthropods. It is also relevant for the patterns of dispersion and efficiency in the transmission of arboviruses by arthropods to their hosts [13]. Considering the perspectives regarding global climate changes, it is likely that arboviruses will continue to colonize new regions of the planet. Thus, research regarding the role of climate in the population dynamics of vectors and predictions of future scenarios depend on the ability of climate-based models to describe associations with arboviruses. Monitoring the effect of climatic variations on vector surveillance and control can be achieved by technological platforms with adequate space time resolution.

This chapter presents two study cases of vector surveillance by sampling egg and adult *Aedes* spp. mosquitoes in Brazilian municipalities. It also provides a comprehensive description of innovative web platforms that process, in near real time, data regarding adult vector abundance and arbovirus identification from mosquitoes caught in sticky traps strategically positioned in urban areas. The information gathered can be used to rapidly activate vector control actions making these platforms successful and cost-effective tools to deal with arboviral disease threats by public health authorities.

2. Gravid mosquito traps

The ovitrap has been used for many decades as a sensitive, inexpensive, passive surveillance tool for detecting the presence of gravid mosquitoes [10, 14]. The addition of a larvicide or autocidal mechanism allows long-term use of ovitraps with minimal risk of the device becoming a productive source of adult mosquitoes [15]. In spite of these positive attributes, ovitraps only provide information on the number of collected eggs and cannot produce accurate information about the number of gravid *Aedes* mosquitoes. This is because a single female can lay different numbers of eggs in a single ovitrap [16], and therefore, information on the presence of eggs alone does not produce enough information about the levels of infestation of a particular area. Another shortcoming of the ovitrap is that it requires laboratory logistics for egg counting, hatching, and identification of the larvae. Consequently, information about the vector population is delayed by at least 1 or 2 weeks [17].

Ovitraps can be modified to collect gravid females by incorporating an adhesive capture surface (sticky ovitraps). Adult female mosquitoes collected in sticky ovitraps provide a direct measure of adult abundance, and those can also be morphologically identified in the field and processed to detect arboviruses [18, 19]. Sampling with sticky ovitraps is a more sensitive method to detect and estimate adult mosquitoes in comparison with sampling of immatures [20–22].

A major advantage of using sticky traps is that the captured mosquitoes can be readily identified in the field at the time of trap inspection. This avoids the need for additional specialized human labor and the delay imposed when samples have to be delivered to laboratories to identify the mosquito [20]. The abundance of adult mosquitoes was successfully estimated in three areas of Rio de Janeiro, Brazil, by using sticky traps [23]. Obviously, these kinds of field-ready results are only possible if field agents are well-trained to identify the mosquito species of *Ae. aegypti*. Indeed, well-trained agents have been shown to accurately (95–100%) identify *Ae. aegypti* captured using the sticky trap MosquiTRAP [24]. However, a later study found that mosquito identification in the laboratory was superior to that performed in locus by trained field agents [25]; divergent results presented by these studies may be due to differences in the way the field agents were trained and qualified.

Several sticky trap models have been developed to capture gravid *Ae. aegypti* in Brazil [20, 26], Australia [18], Italy [27], Porto Rico [28], and Malaysia [29]. All rely on a combination of visual and olfactory stimuli for the oviposition behavior of gravid *Aedes* spp. Typically, a sticky trap consists of a black matte plastic container of any size, an entrance port, water, an oviposition attractant, and a sticky card using an odorless entomological glue to retain the gravid mosquito. Once stuck, the mosquito remains in resting position. Those that escape usually loose one or more legs remain adhered to the sticky card. Identification of collected mosquitoes is still possible with their thoraces since they usually remain somewhat visible [18, 20]. Sticky traps do not require electricity or batteries and are, therefore, low-cost devices.

The oviposition attractants include infusions of organic materials such as hay [15], grass infusions [30], or synthetic lures [31]. The chemical composition of synthetic oviposition attractants was derived from research that identified volatiles of grass infusions that were behaviorally active in laboratory, semi-field, and field studies. The synthetic oviposition attractant Atr*Aedes*™ used in the MosquiTRAP consists of a mixture of nonanal, decanal, and 3-methylphenol, which is released from a sealed-tube reservoir system for approximately 45 days at a constant rate to continually attract the target species [31]. The main advantage of using synthetic attractants is that the synthetic lure has a constant attractiveness over time and has a pleasant smell, whereas grass infusions need to be transported and rest for 5–7 days to be active and are smelly.

The place where the sticky trap is positioned in the investigated premises is important to increase the mosquito catch rate. Studies in Brazil revealed that when the sticky trap MosquiTRAP was placed outdoor, it captured five times more females than indoor traps [26]. This is probably because host-seeking *Ae. aegypti* feed on human blood indoors but lay eggs outdoors after a few days of digesting the blood meal. Moreover, outdoor traps allow vector control workers to sample the mosquitoes without inconveniencing homeowners and are notably well-accepted by local communities [17, 18, 27, 32].

The potential of the MosquiTRAP for trapping gravid *Ae. aegypti* has been compared with the Nasci aspirator [33] and backpack aspirator [34]. Sticky traps collected a higher number of mosquitoes and are more cost-effective and operationally easier, besides being less inconvenient to householders than active traps. MosquiTRAP has ben also compared with BG-Sentinel trap and Adultrap and ovitrap with favorable results [35].

Altogether, sticky traps are perhaps the most appropriate tools for *Ae. aegypti* surveillance and the development of new entomological indices for the detection of epidemic outbreaks in urban areas. Interestingly, a study comparing the ability to detect *Ae. aegypti* by the different surveillance methods (larval survey, ovitrap, and the sticky trap MosquiTRAP) showed that ovitrap and the sticky trap predicted dengue occurrence better than larval survey, both spatially and temporally. However, ovitrap clusters showed less accuracy in pinpointing the dengue risk areas, and the sticky trap presented better results for signaling dengue transmission risk both geographically and temporally (**Figure 3**) [36].

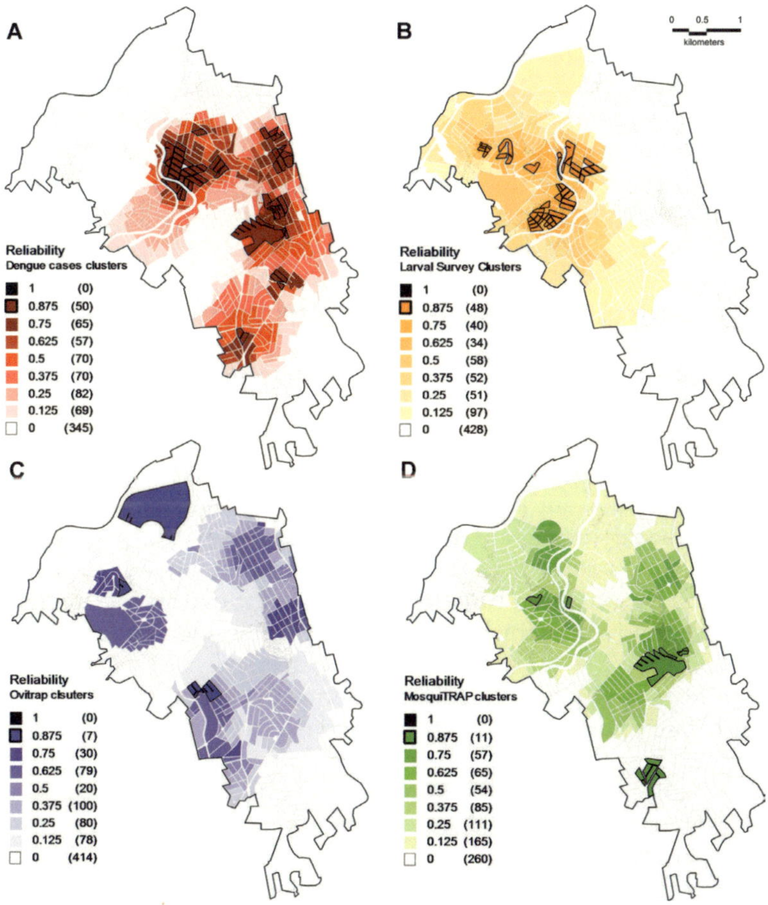

Figure 3.
Cluster reliability maps of (A) dengue cases, (B) larval survey, (C) ovitrap, and (D) MosquiTRAP catches in Belo Horizonte (Minas Gerais, Brazil) from January 2007 to June 2008. Darker colors represent higher reliability values (Belo Horizonte city, Minas Gerais State, Brazil, Adapted from De Melo et al. [36]).

3. Use of geographic information system (GIS) for vector surveillance

GIS is a powerful automated system for the capture, storage, retrieval, analysis, and display of spatial data that offer expanding opportunities for epidemiology because it allows a spatial perspective on a disease. The integration of vector surveillance with the mosquito traps and georeferencing technologies has emerged as an important tool for fighting *Ae. aegypti* and transmission of arboviruses [31, 37, 38].

By georeferencing the ovitrap and sticky traps, the egg collection and adult catching data obtained during *Ae. aegypti* surveillance was used to generate maps that show the areas of high and low infestation [31, 39–42]. This information provides real-time data and allows spatial analyses to determine vector control actions and to evaluate their impact on mosquito populations and infection with arboviruses [31, 39, 43]. The continuous surveillance of *Aedes* population allied with mathematical modeling strategies (described below) allows reliable predictions of infestation, as shown in Brazil [12].

4. Brazilian case studies

Two types of traps associated with georeferencing systems were developed and evaluated continuously in Brazil: (1) ovitraps associated with the surveillance platform MSCP-*Aedes* (Monitoring System and Population Control for urban *Aedes*) and (2) sticky traps for gravid *Aedes* mosquitoes associated with a real-time, large-scale surveillance system known as MI-*Aedes* platform (from Portuguese "Monitoramento Integrado do *Aedes*"). Both systems will be described below, with emphasis on the adult trapping technology—MI-*Aedes*—since it has been used in the last 13 years in hundreds of Brazilian cities.

4.1 Monitoring system and population control for urban *Aedes* (MSCP-*Aedes*)

The MSCP-*Aedes* platform was developed by the National Institute for Space Research (INPE) and Research Center Aggeu Magalhães (CPqAM), Oswaldo Cruz Foundation (Fiocruz), located in Recife city, Pernambuco State, Brazil. The potential of ovitraps in reducing the population of *Aedes* spp. was evaluated for 1 year (April 2014–April 2015), during all seasons of the year (summer, autumn, winter, and spring), by the deployment of 464 georeferenced traps in five areas of Recife, the capital city of the state of Pernambuco, located in northeastern Brazil. Thirteen egg collection cycles were performed with 98.5% of the ovitraps being positive for *Aedes* eggs. At the end of the study, more than 4 million eggs were collected from the environment, and the *Ae. aegypti* population in one of the five localities evaluated was significantly reduced. The platform provided information on the spatial-temporal distribution of *Aedes* spp. eggs. Using this data, maps generated within a GIS environment helped the health authorities to prioritize the city areas in most need of vector control actions [40] (**Figure 4**).

Another pilot trial of the MSCP-*Aedes* system was carried out from March 2008 to October 2011 in two other cities of Pernambuco State, Brazil: Ipojuca and Santa Cruz [37]. After the first 2 years of evaluation, a significant decrease in the density of eggs was observed in both cities showing the potential of the MSCP-*Aedes* platform associated with the vector control actions conducted by the health authorities to reduce mosquito abundance (**Figure 5**). However, the MSCP-*Aedes* platform required a great number of people to accomplish the field and laboratory activities, which is not realistic to use in a large-scale scenario.

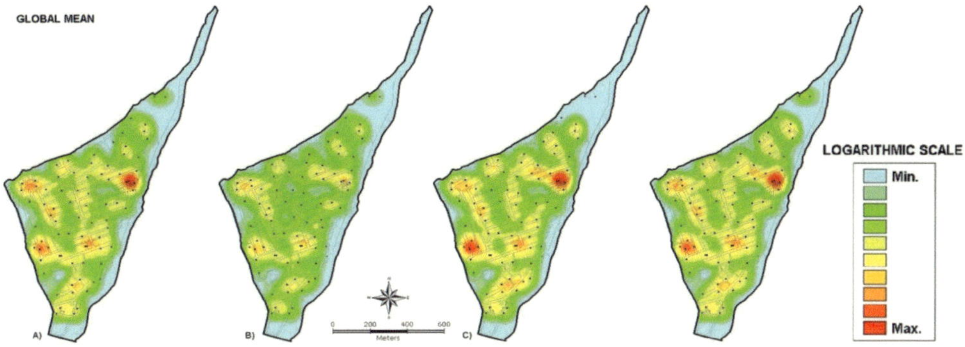

Figure 4.
Spatial distribution of Aedes spp. eggs in Brasília Teimosa (Recife, Pernambuco State, Brazil), in June–July 2004 (A), December 2004 (B), and March 2005 (C). Green, low infestation; yellow, intermediate infestation; red, high infestation. The map at the right shows the mean number of eggs for the whole period (April 2004 to April 2005). Adapted from Regis et al. [40].

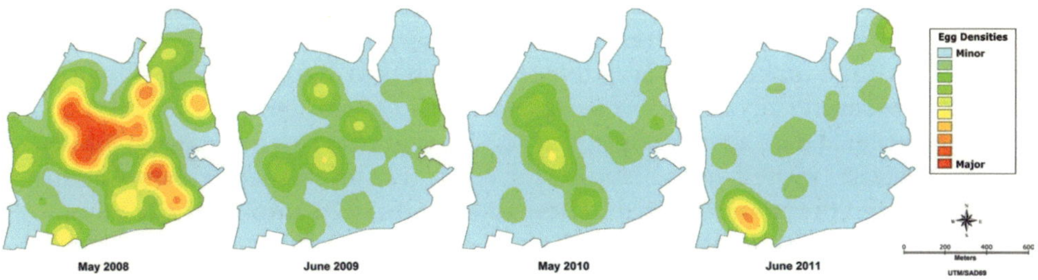

Figure 5.
Spatial distribution of Aedes eggs at the high-density period (May–June) in Ipojuca (Recife, Brazil), Pernambuco State, 2008–2011. The mass suppression of eggs using 2700 control ovitraps started in October 2009 (Adapted from Regis et al. [37]).

4.2 Integrated *Aedes* surveillance system (MI-*Aedes*)

The innovative MI-*Aedes* platform was developed in Brazil by a university-company partnership between the Federal University of Minas Gerais and the university's "spin-off" Ecovec, in Belo Horizonte, Minas Gerais State. University-Company partnerships have been stimulated by the Brazilian Innovation Law, which aims to foster the generation of innovations and dissemination of new technologies aiming to solve national (and international) problems [44, 45]. The World Health Organization has praised this new technology for the surveillance and generation of entomological indices [46]. More details about the platform are given below.

The MI-*Aedes* platform consists of (a) the sticky trap MosquiTRAP (baited with a Atr*Aedes* to generate mosquito abundance indices), which is placed within blocks of urban areas 250 m equidistant from each other and inspected weekly, (b) the recording of entomological data on electronic spreadsheets or by cell phone during trap inspection, and (c) an Internet site that integrates real-time adult mosquito surveillance data and GIS technology to provide entomological indices [12, 31, 36, 38, 41, 47, 48] (**Figure 6**).

The information used for vector control relies on (1) weekly surveillance of gravid *Ae. aegypti* infestation of the municipality street blocks, (2) re-infestation surveillance of the monitored blocks, (3) identification of hotspot areas, and (4) production of entomological indices.

The MI-*Aedes* Web-data system consists of three integrated software developed to simplify information gathering and processing: (a) the "'geo-mosquito

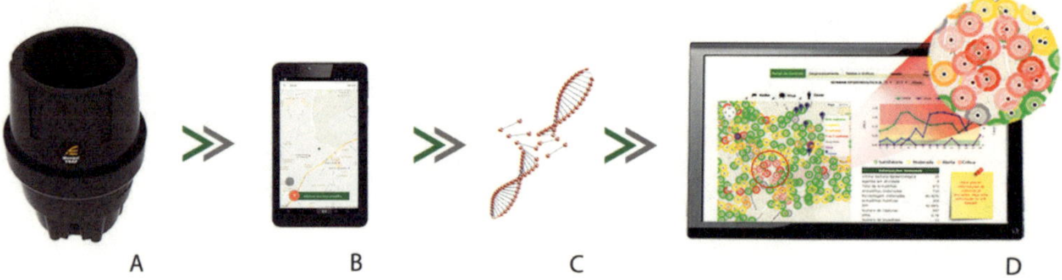

Figure 6.
The MI-Aedes platform consists of (A) sticky trap (MosquiTRAP), (B) cell phone for sampling GIS mosquito data, (C) MI-Virus (optional—see text for detail), and (D) Internet georeferenced maps at real time that produces automatic data for entomological indices.

collection," which is installed in portable devices (e.g., cell phones) to record household information, placement of the trap within the residence, and *Ae. aegypti* field capture data; (b) the "monitoring," which processes the field data to produce tables with entomological indices and graphs showing trends; and (c) the "geo-*Aedes*," which produces georeferenced maps of mosquitoes captured with the sticky MosquiTRAP and makes them available to users on the Internet on a weekly basis.

There are several advantages of using electronic spreadsheets or mobile phone over conventional data acquisition systems. The field data can be accessed immediately (premises visited and scheduled for visits, trap locations, residents' names, and so on), and the entomological indices can be produced automatically. Also, there is no delay between the data that is reported to the database and the database that is available for web mapping and public health access.

The MI-*Aedes* platform was evaluated in hundreds of Brazilian cities for more than 10 years and showed to greatly reduce arbovirus transmission [41]. The georeferenced maps presented weekly on the Internet by the MI-*Aedes* platform allowed health managers to identify the infestation status of city blocks by the colors green, yellow, orange, and red, according to the number of adult *Ae. aegypti* females captured (**Figure 7**). The weekly data evaluating vector infestation levels became an important information for dengue control programs because it helped public health managers to optimize *Ae. aegypti* control activities with improved precision of the target activities to the infested blocks. Indeed, a study analyzing three Brazilian municipalities revealed that following implementation of the MI-*Aedes* platform, the weekly vector control indicator established by the entomological "mean female *Aedes* index "(MFAI) was reduced (**Figure 7**) and so was the number of dengue cases [31]. Further research showed how the health authorities used the platform to evaluate the performance of the control measures employed by them within the area covered by the MI-*Aedes* [12, 41].

4.2.1 Virus detection of trapped gravid Aedes spp. collected by the sticky trap MosquiTRAP

The detection of gravid mosquitoes infected with arboviruses such as DENV, CHIKV, and ZIKV is an important information for public health managers looking to control *Ae. aegypti* infestation and the spread of arboviral diseases in hotspot areas. The inclusion of a strategy to identify the arbovirus present in infected mosquitoes trapped in the MosquiTRAP into the MI-*Aedes* platform was intended to provide additional information regarding the spread of arboviruses and serve as an early warning system for epidemics since viral detection in mosquitoes can precede detection in humans. Accordingly, a rapid and well-established method for arbovirus identification [49] was associated with the MI-*Aedes* platform to create an

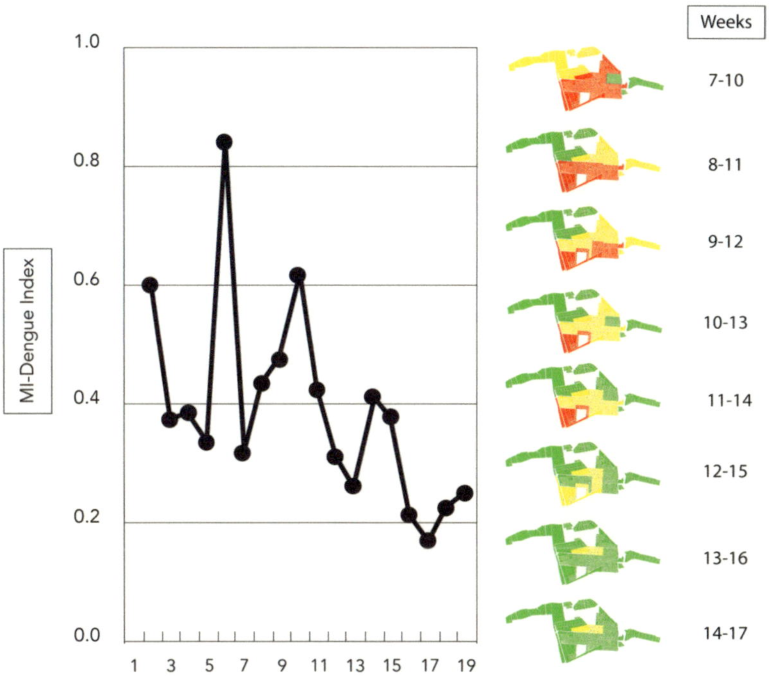

Figure 7.
Temporal and spatial analysis of neighborhoods in the municipality of Presidente Epitácio (São Paulo State, Brazil) (2008). Colored maps are classified according to the entomological indices from epidemiological week 7–16 (February–April, summer). In epidemiological weeks 7–10, there were 44 and 55% of neighborhoods classified as "dengue alert" and "critical," respectively. Weeks 14–17 were 88.9 and 11.1% of the municipality's territory as "risk-free" and "dengue alert," respectively, indicating a strong seasonal variation in the Aedes aegypti population density that was probably influenced by the climate conditions or targeted control measures. Adapted from Eiras and Resende [31].

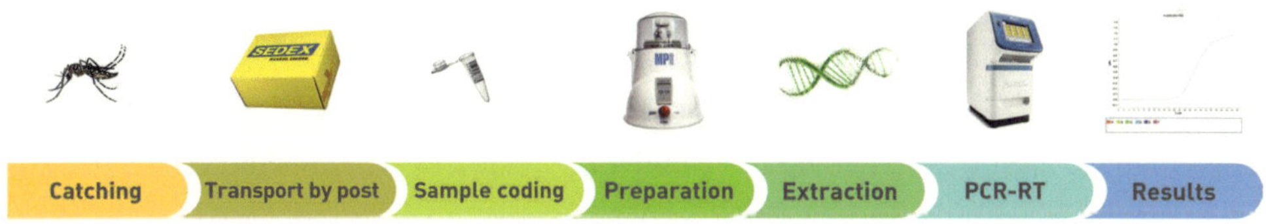
Catching
Transport by post
Sample coding
Preparation
Extraction
PCR-RT
Results

Figure 8.
Logistic of the Integrated Monitoring Virus (MI-Virus). Weekly, caught female Aedes aegypti by MosquiTRAP are place in barcoded Eppendorf tube and send by post to laboratory for RT-PCR analysis. Bar code provides GIS trap position. Source: Ecovec Company, Belo Horizonte, Minas Gerais State, Brazil.

Integrated Monitoring Virus (MI-Virus) platform. The trapped *Ae. aegypti* and *Ae. albopictus* are placed in Eppendorf tubes with guanidine and sent by mail for virus detection and identification by reverse transcriptase RT-PCR (**Figure 8**).

In Brazil, the MI-Virus platform was tested in hundreds of municipalities to detect and map not only *Ae. aegypti* abundance but also the presence of mosquito populations infected with different arboviruses such as DENV, CHIKV, and ZIKV. The use of MosquiTRAP to detect DENV-infected gravid *Ae. aegypti* trapped by was performed in Brazil [41, 50] and Colombia [51]. In In 2017, the MI-*Aedes* and MI-Virus platforms were used during an outbreak of chikungunya in Governador Valadares city, located in the southeastern state of Minas Gerais, Brazil (data not published). The real-time data obtained by the MI-*Aedes* platform and the confirmation of CHIKV by the MI-Virus (**Figure 9**) led the health authorities to act quickly and employ additional vector control activities to target areas with the

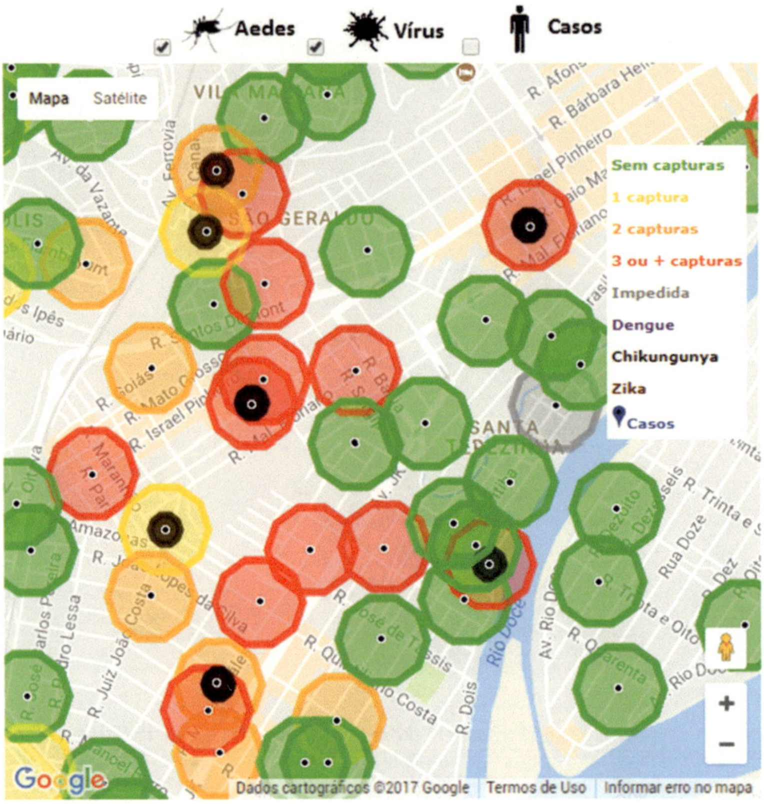

Figure 9.
Data obtained by the MI-Aedes platform and MI-Virus deployed in Governador Valadares city, Minas Gerais State, Brazil (epidemiological week 11, March 05–11, 2017). Dark dots at colored circles mean MosquiTRAP (GIS) position. Colored circles mean infestation status of mosquito abundance (see text for further detail). Black circles mean infected Aedes aegypti by chikungunya virus captured by MosquiTRAP (data not published). Source: Ecovec company, Belo Horizonte, Minas Gerais State, Brazil.

highest mosquito densities. As a result, abundance of *Ae. aegypti* and chikungunya cases reduced significantly (data not published). Futures studies should be conducted of arbovirus detections in other areas.

4.2.2 Modeling the population dynamics of Aedes aegypti using MI-Aedes

Once vector surveillance and control are established as the recommended approach to manage vector-borne diseases, the ecological problem of the population dynamics of mosquitoes arises as a fundamental question [52]. In such context, mathematical modeling has a twofold role: to assist the validation of these novel technologies by providing methods to predict the population dynamics of adult mosquitoes and to offer ways to improve the surveillance indices. As an ecological problem, the infestation by mosquitoes is influenced by many anthropic (everything that results from human action such as sanitation and mosquito breeding container) and non-anthropic variables (temperature and rainfall) [53]. It has been well established that the population dynamics of different stages of *Ae. aegypti* and viral transmission are influenced by environmental variables, especially those of climate: temperature, humidity, and precipitation [54–58]. The vector-virus-human system can generate multiple sources of complexity for modeling. The vector management approach of considering the female population as a risk of infection indicator helps to simplify the modeling efforts, which can decouple the complex ecological vector-virus-human system and focus on the mosquito population. In addition, the surveillance platform MI-*Aedes* generates a huge amount of sampling data from many localities [12, 59, 60]. These huge data banks provided basis for many modeling studies such as a novel stochastic point process pattern algorithm that identify the spatial and temporal association between DENV-infected mosquitoes and human cases. This process showed a strong and significant association between high DENV incidence in mosquitoes and the onset of symptoms in humans at specific spatial and temporal windows [61]. Also the model goodness-of-fit studies based on the number of sticky traps and suggests a minimum of 16 traps for the MI-*Aedes* at the neighborhood level for mosquito surveillance [62].

Decades of studies regarding the effects of temperature, precipitation, and humidity on vector population and the occurrence of infectious disease cases generated controversial conclusions, suggesting that the phenomenon depends on local specificities, as extensively demonstrated for dengue [54, 63]. Nevertheless, it is well established that temperature affects the physiology of the mosquito and virus and, consequently, is associated with the vector population size and dengue cases [13, 58, 64–66]. Humidity greatly affects the development of vector stages and the number of dengue infections [67, 68]. Although precipitation is strongly correlated with humidity, due to its complex pattern and unpredictable influence in the environment, it figures as the most complex meteorological variable [69]. Notwithstanding, precipitation is a good explanatory variable for dengue cases and mosquito population size [70]. Hence, the construction of models to explain the effects of climatological variables cannot disregard the complete set of these influential variables.

The problem of describing or even predicting a response time series such as disease cases or infestation can be approached with descriptive models, which provide a model time series solution by fitting coefficients and/or functions in accordance with past lagged time series of a set of explanatory variables. Belonging to that class are the regressive models, which have been used for predicting or describing the number of dengue cases or the degree of adult *Ae. aegypti* infestation [12, 56, 59, 71]. Through a descriptive model, time series of temperature, precipitation, wind velocity, and humidity were analyzed as explanatory variables for the adult mosquito abundance index MFAI in the subhumid tropical climate of the city of Governador Valadares, Brazil [59]. In the study, generalized linear models (GLM) with time lags and interaction terms between explanatory variables were used to identify the following significant associations: interaction between lagged temperature and humidity with the mosquito abundance data obtained on the previous week. Transient associations were mapped in a periodogram using wavelets and revealed significant effects for precipitation and wind velocity. Interestingly, the wavelet technique identified non-stationary effects on the relationship between meteorological variables and infestation.

Another study using descriptive models was conducted in the city of Porto Alegre, located in a humid subtropical region of southern Brazil. It used data derived from monitoring the *Ae. aegypti* adult female population in the course of MI-Dengue (nowadays, MI-*Aedes*) surveillance platform [12]. As described above, the platform employs sticky traps to capture adult *Ae. aegypti* females to provide a weekly infestation index. To predict mosquito abundance in subsequent weeks, time series data from previous weeks regarding the maximum, minimum, and mean temperature, precipitation, humidity, and mosquito abundance were fitted in a set of proposed models using generalized additive models (GAM). The best power of prediction was achieved when previous values of minimum temperatures and adult females were included in the set of explanatory variables (**Figure 10**). Precipitation was not a significant explanatory variable for the humid temperate climate of Porto

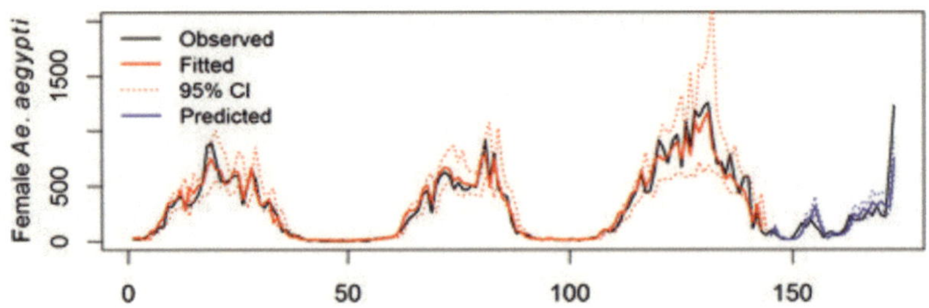

Figure 10.
Observed adult infestation index MFAI and predicted generalized additive models (GAM) with meteorological and infestation data as explanatory variables for the city of Porto Alegre, Rio Grande do Sul, Brazil. From September 2012 to January 2016 (Figure extracted from da Cruz Ferreira et al. [12]).

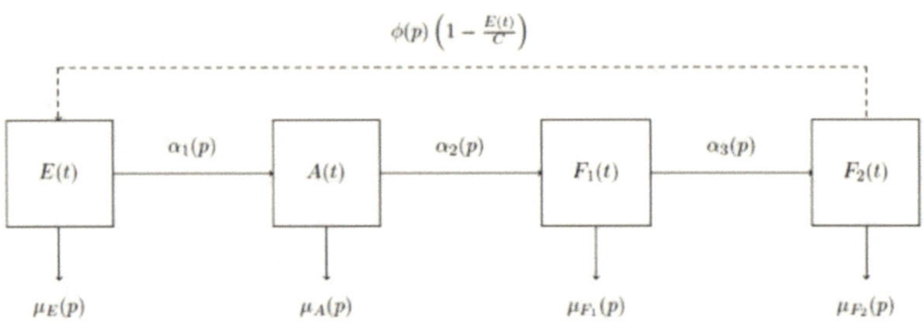

Figure 11.
Mechanistic model comprising the populations of the stages of development of Aedes aegypti: E(t), A(t), F1(t), and F2(t), which are the populations of eggs, aquatic forms, and females pre and post blood meal, respectively. The rates of development of the model are set to depend on precipitation p. The curves are generated after solving a system of nonlinear differential equations, the preferred framework to represent that class of models (data not published).

Alegre, presumably because precipitation is less seasonal in this region. The association between mosquito infestation and the number of dengue cases was positive, indicating that the infestation index MFAI is a good indicator for the risk of arboviral transmission [12].

Mechanistic models have the same goal of describing or even predicting a time response series as the descriptive models but differ from the latter because they are structured with realism based on the natural phenomena, for example, the population model comprises the biological cycle of *Ae. aegypti*. Hence, through these models, from deviations and corrections for adjustment to the data, it is possible to reveal the cause-effect relations of the underlying phenomena.

Mechanistic models have been used to study and predict vector infestation and the number of dengue cases [60, 72–78]. One such model was developed to account for the effect of precipitation on the stages of development of *Ae. aegypti* by setting the model parameters as dependent on the precipitation index (in millimeters) (**Figure 11**) [60]. **Figure 12** illustrates the model result considering the infestation index MFAI and the precipitation from June 2009 to December 2010 for the city of Sete Lagoas, Minas Gerais, Brazil.

4.2.3 Cost-benefit of the MI-Aedes platform

Dengue epidemics pose a heavy burden on health services and the economy of any country. Recently, studies in eight countries in the Americas and Asia have shown that the cost of epidemics in these countries reached approximately US$ 1.8 billion per year [79, 80]. This number only refers to the money spent on outpatient and hospital expenses and did not consider costs such as those related to

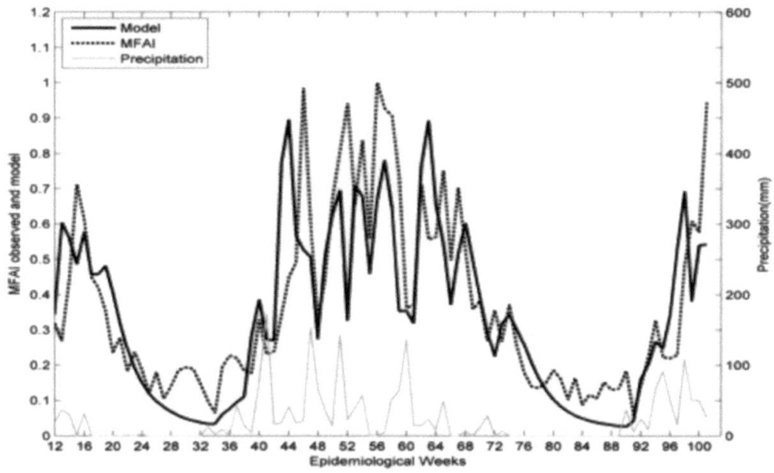

Figure 12.
Comparison of 83 epidemiological weeks covering the time series data of Aedes aegypti females captured divided by the number of traps (MFAI), the model result, and the precipitation index in the municipality of Sete Lagoas, Minas Gerais, Brazil. From June 2009 to December 2010 (J.L. Acebal—data not published).

surveillance and vector control activities. The economic losses imposed by arboviral diseases involve the patient's withdrawal from productive activities, drug expenses, hospitalization, medical consultations, treatment of sequelae, and death [81]. The time needed to treat and recover from arboviruses varies. On average, dengue removes the affected patient for 10–12 days from their work activities. The ZIKV may lead to birth defects including microcephaly and other severe brain malformations, which impose lifetime incapacity. Recovery from chikungunya varies from months to years [82].

Following the guidelines of the National Program for Dengue Control (PNCD), the MI-*Aedes* and MI-Virus technologies were adopted by the health authorities of the state of Minas Gerais (Brazil) and implemented in 21 cities with a high incidence of dengue in the period 2009–2011. The total cost of the program for all 21 cities for 2 years of work was less than US$ 1.5 million, making an average of US$ 71,428 per city. It included 4700 sticky traps, 115,000 sticky cards, synthetic oviposition attractants, RT-PCR on all mosquitoes caught in the traps, Web software licensing, cell phones, and technical support, among other items. The number of people benefited by the program was approximately 2 million, making the cost per habitant per year around US$ 0.70. The cost-effectiveness was calculated as the cost of running the MI-*Aedes* and MI-Virus platforms divided by the number of cases of prevented arboviral diseases compared with cities that did not use the MI-*Aedes* platform and relied only in the PNCD guidelines. The MI-*Aedes* and MI-Virus platforms prevented a total of 27,191 cases at a total cost of US$ 7.5 million, thus saving approximately US$ 0.4 million in direct costs (health care and vector control) and US$ 7.1 million in lost wages (societal impact) annually [41]. The cost-effectiveness of the platforms MI-*Aedes* and MI-Virus in cities with high mosquito infestation levels emphasizes the power of using these new technologies in vector control practices.

Currently, the MI-*Aedes* platform is running simultaneously in 154 Brazilian cities targeting approximately 7.5 million people, using about 12,000 sticky traps, and performing 625,000 trap inspections and around 8200 RT-PCR analysis per month on pooled mosquitoes (source: Ecovec. Ltd).

Investing more effort into integrating MI-*Aedes* strategies and costs with vector control operations, and standardizing the MI-*Aedes*-based control system across cities, should help to increase the platform cost-effectiveness. Future studies should be conducted for developing new predictive model of serotype dynamics across cities for accurate arboviruses transmission.

5. Conclusions

In Brazil, two platforms for surveillance of eggs and gravid *Aedes aegypti* have been developed. First, the use of gravid traps associated with GIS technologies was used in Brazil in the last years to monitor *Aedes* spp. populations. The MSCP-*Aedes* platform is based on data collected upon sampling of eggs in ovitrap works. Although effective, the platform requires a large amount of human resources for field and laboratory activities that is not realistic to use in a large-scale epidemic scenario.

Second, the MI-*Aedes* and MI-Virus platforms described herein have been used in hundreds of cities and in a variety of scales besides of being a cost-effective (less than US$ 1.00/person/year) approach to reduce mosquito population and prevent the transmission of arbovirosis such as dengue, chikungunya, and Zika [13, 41]. The main advantage of the MI-*Aedes* platform over traditional mosquito surveillance is the integration of continuous vector monitoring at fine spatial and temporal scales coupled to an information technology platform for near real-time data collection, analysis, and decision-making.

The surveillance data generated with the MI-*Aedes* platform is used to calculate weekly vector indices and detect hotspots to help health authorities to strategically manage vector control resources. The platform is suitable to be implemented at worldwide scale because it does not require extensive infrastructure or expertise. For example, one field surveillance agent can visit 70–100 traps per week, conduct mosquito identification, and feed the database using a cell phone. More importantly, the MI-*Aedes* platform is the only large-scale mosquito surveillance system with a good track record on the prevention of cases of dengue [41]. Used to their optimum level, as tools for analysis and decision-making, the MI-*Aedes* and MI-Virus platforms are information management vehicles with high public health potential. Indeed, it is worth mentioning that this platform not only provides a wide range of GIS tools for *Ae. aegypti* surveillance, but the data collection and processing modules can be adapted to monitor other diseases, such as AIDS, tuberculosis, malaria, and leishmaniosis, among others.

6. Future studies

Studies with MI-*Aedes* platform should be continuously conducted to improve the accuracy and threshold of arbovirus outbreaks. The sensitivity of trap device of the MI-Aedes platform will be enhanced by replacing the MosquiTRAP by the GAT as it has been shown to be more effective [11]. Currently, studies using MI-*Aedes* and MI-Virus technologies for monitoring vector and virus circulation (DENV, CHIKV, and ZIKV) together with new mathematical models are very important tools to address targeted areas for vector control address. Future studies using MI-Aedes platform in association with integrated mosquito control alternatives, such as *Wolbachia* and transgenic mosquitoes, should be also conducted. Those combinations of interventions will be best applied in sustained, proactive implementation and will likely be suitable for rapid control of a developing epidemic. In addition to such proactive strategies, arbovirus prevention will benefit from greater capacity for outbreak response, before outbreaks have peaked and begun to decline on their own.

Acknowledgements

AEE acknowledges the Brazilian funding agencies CNPq, FINEP, FAPEMIG, CAPES, SVS-MS, and SCTIE-MS. KSP thanks the fellowships from CAPES and CNPq and USAID. The authors thank Ecovec for providing additional information of MI-Aedes platform and Pedro Lassis for the creation of figures of the technologies.

Conflict of interest

The authors claim no conflict of interest.

List of abbreviations

AGO	Autocidal Gravid Ovitrap
AIDS	acquired immunodeficiency syndrome
CDC	Centers for Disease Control and Prevention
CHIKV	chikungunya virus
CPqAM	Research Center Aggeu Magalhães
DENV	dengue virus
Fiocruz	Oswaldo Cruz Foundation
GAM	generalized additive models
GAT	Gravid *Aedes* Trap
GIS	geographic information system
GLM	generalized linear models
INPE	National Institute for Space Research
MFAI	mean female *Aedes* index
MI-*Aedes*	from Portuguese "Monitoramento Integrado do *Aedes*"
MI-Dengue	from Portuguese "Monitoramento Inteligente da Dengue"
MI-Virus	integrated monitoring of virus
MSCP-*Aedes*	monitoring system and population control for urban *Aedes*
PNCD	National Program for Dengue Control
RT-PCR	reverse transcription polymerase chain reaction
ZIKV	Zika virus

Author details

Alvaro E. Eiras[1*], Marcelo C. Resende[1,2], José L. Acebal[3] and Kelly S. Paixão[1]

1 Department of Parasitology, Biological Sciences Institute, Federal University of Minas Gerais, Belo Horizonte, MG, Brazil

2 National Health Foundation, Ministry of Health, Belo Horizonte, MG, Brazil

3 Department of Physics and Mathematics, Federal Centre for Technological Education of Minas Gerais, Belo Horizonte, MG, Brazil

*Address all correspondence to: alvaro@icb.ufmg.br

References

[1] Kraemer MUG, Sinka ME, Duda KA, Mylne AQN, Shearer FM, Barker CM, et al. The global distribution of the arbovirus vectors *Aedes aegypti* and *Ae. albopictus*. eLife. 2015;**4**:e08347. DOI: 10.7554/eLife.08347.002

[2] Norris DE. Mosquito-borne diseases as a consequence of land use change. EcoHealth. 2004;**1**(1):19-24

[3] Simmons CP, Farrar JJ, Chau NV, Wills B. Dengue. The New England Journal of Medicine. 2012;**366**:1423-1432

[4] Jentes ES, Poumero G, Gershman MD, Hill DR, Johan Lemarchand J, Rosamund FLewis RJ, et al. The revised global yellow fever risk map and recommendations for vaccination, 2010: Consensus of the informal WHO working group on geographic risk for yellow fever. The Lancet. Infectious Diseases. 2011;**11**:622-632

[5] Leparc-Goffart, Nougairede A, Cassadou S, Prat C, de Lamballerie X. Chikungunya in the Americas. Lancet. 2014;**383**:514

[6] Messina JP, Kraemer MUG, Brady OJ, Pigott DM, Shearer FM, Weiss DJ, et al. Mapping global environmental suitability for Zika virus. Epidemiology and global health microbiology and infectious disease. eLife. 2016;**5**:e15272. DOI: 10.7554/eLife.15272

[7] Brady OJ, Gething PW, Bhatt S, Messina JP, Brownstein JS, Hoen AG, et al. Refining the global spatial limits of dengue virus transmission by evidence-based consensus. PLoS Neglected Tropical Diseases. 2012;**6**:e1760

[8] Bhatt S, Gething PW, Brady OJ, Messina JP, Farlow AW, Moyes CL, et al. The global distribution and burden of dengue. Nature. 2013;**496**:504-507

[9] Organización Panamericana de la Salud [Internet]. Zika- Actualización epidemiológica; 21 de abril del 2016; [1 p.]. Washington (DC): OPS. Disponible en: http://www.paho.org/hq/index.php?option=com_docman&task=doc_view&Itemid=270&gid=34245&lang=es

[10] Fay RW, Eliason DA. A preferred oviposition site as surveillance method for *Aedes aegypti*. Mosquito News. 1966;**26**:531-535

[11] Johnson JJ, Ritchie SA, Fonseca DM. The state of the art of lethal oviposition trap-based mass interventions for arboviral control. Insects. 2017;**8**:5. DOI: 10.3390/insects8010005

[12] Da Cruz Ferreira DA, Degener CM, Marques-Toledo C, Bendati MM, Fetzer LO, Teixeira CP, et al. Meteorological variables and mosquito monitoring are good predictors for infestation trends of *Aedes aegypti*, the vector of dengue, chikungunya and Zika. Parasites & Vectors. 2017;**10**:78-91

[13] Chowell G, Sanchez F. Climate-based descriptive models of dengue fever: The 2002 epidemic in Colima, Mexico. Journal of Environmental Health. 2006;**68**(10):40

[14] World Health Organization. Entomological Surveillance for *Aedes* spp. in the Context of Zika Virus. Interim guidance for entomologists [Internet]. 2016. WHO/ZIKV/VC/16.2. Available from: http://apps.who.int/iris/bitstream/10665/204624/1/WHO_ZIKV_VC_16.2_eng.pdf [Accessed: December 12, 2017]

[15] Perich M, Kardec A, Braga I, Portal I, Burge R, Zeichner B, et al. Field evaluation of a lethal ovitrap against dengue vectors in Brazil. Medical and Veterinary Entomology. 2003;**17**:205-210

[16] Abreu FVS, Morais MM, Ribeiro SP, Eiras AE. Influence of breeding site availability on the oviposition behaviour of *Aedes aegypti*. Memórias do Instituto Oswaldo Cruz. 2015;**110**(5):669-676. DOI: 10.1590/0074-02760140490

[17] Resende MC, Silva IM, Ellis BR, Eiras AE. A comparison of larval, ovitrap and MosquiTRAP surveillance for *Aedes (Stegomyia) aegypti*. Memórias do Instituto Oswaldo Cruz. 2013;**108**(8):1024-1030

[18] Ritchie SA, Long S, Hart A, Webb C, Russell RC. An adulticidal sticky ovitrap for sampling container-breeding mosquitoes. Journal of the American Mosquito Control Association. 2003;**19**:235-242. DOI: 10.1590/0074-0276130128

[19] Vilela APP, Figueiredo LB, dos Santos JR, Eiras AE, Bonjardim CA, Ferreira PCP, et al. Dengue virus 3 genotype I in *Aedes aegypti* mosquitoes and eggs, Brazil, 2005-2006. Emerging Infectious Diseases. 2010;**16**(6):989-992. DOI: 10.3201/eid1606.091000

[20] Gama RA, Silva EM, Silva IM, Resende MC, Eiras AE. Evaluation of the sticky MosquiTRAP for detecting *Aedes (Stegomyia) aegypti* (L.) (Diptera: Culicidae) during the dry season in Belo Horizonte, Minas Gerais, Brazil. Neotropical Entomology. 2007;**36**:294-902. DOI: 10.1590/S1519-566X2007000200018

[21] Honório NA, Nogueira RMR, Codeço CT, Carvalho MS, Cruz OG, Magalhães MAFM, et al. Spatial evaluation and modeling of dengue seroprevalence and vector density in Rio de Janeiro, Brazil. PLoS Neglected Tropical Diseases. 2009;**3**(11):e545. DOI: 10.1371/journal.pntd.0000545

[22] Steffler LM, Marteis LS, Dolabella SS, Cavalcanti SCH, dos Santos RC. Risk of dengue occurrence based on the capture of gravid *Aedes aegypti* females using MosquiTRAP. Memórias do Instituto Oswaldo Cruz. 2011;**106**(3):365-367. DOI: 10.1590/S0074-02762011000300018

[23] Honório N, Codeço CT, Alves FC Magalhães MAFM, Lourenço-de-Oliveira R. Temporal distribution of *Aedes aegypti* in different districts of Rio de Janeiro, Brazil, measured by two types of traps. Journal of Medical Entomology. 2009;**46**(5):1001-1014

[24] Resende MC, Silva IM, Eiras AE. Avaliação da operacionalidade da armadilha MosquiTRAP no monitoramento de *Aedes aegypti*. Epidemiologia e Serviços de Saúde. 2010;**19**:329-338

[25] Maciel-de-Freitas R, Lima AWS, Araújo SC, Lima JBP, Galardo AKR, Honório NA, et al. Discrepancies between *Aedes aegypti* identification in the field and in the laboratory after collection with a sticky trap. Memórias do Instituto Oswaldo Cruz. 2014;**109**:824-827

[26] Fávaro EA, Dibo MR, Mondini A, Ferreira AC, Barbosa AC, Eiras AE, et al. Physiological state of *Aedes (Stegomyia) aegypti* mosquitoes captured with MosquiTRAPs™ in Mirassol, São Paulo, Brazil. Journal of Vector Ecology. 2006;**31**(2):285-291. DOI: 10.3376/1081-1710(2006)31[285:PSOASA]2.0.CO;2

[27] Facchinelli L, Valerio L, Pombi M, Reiter P, Constantini C, Della Torre A. Development of a novel sticky trap for container-breeding mosquitoes and evaluation of its sampling properties to monitor urban populations of *Aedes albopictus*. Medical and Veterinary Entomology. 2007;**21**:183-195

[28] Mackay AJ, Amador M, Barrera R. An improved autocidal gravid ovitrap for the control and surveillance of *Aedes aegypti*. Parasites & Vectors. 2013;**6**:225. DOI: 10.1186/1756-3305-6-225

[29] Roslan MA, Ngui R, Vythilingam I, Sulaiman WYW. Evaluation of sticky traps for adult *Aedes* mosquitoes in Malaysia: A potential monitoring and surveillance tool for the efficacy of control strategies. Journal of Vector Ecology. 2017;**42**(2):298-307. DOI: 10.1111/jvec.12270

[30] Sant'Ana AL, Roque RA, Eiras AE. Characteristics of grass infusions as oviposition attractants to (Diptera: Culicidae). Journal of Medical Entomology. 2006;**43**:214-220

[31] Eiras AE, Resende MC. Preliminary evaluation of the "Dengue-MI" technology for *Aedes aegypti* monitoring and control. Cadernos de Saúde Pública. 2009;**25**(Sup. 1):S45-S58. DOI: 10.1590/S0102-311X2009001300005

[32] Ordónez-Gonzalez JG, Mercado-Hernandez R, Florez-Suarez AE, Fernandez-Salas I. The use of sticky ovitraps to estimate dispersal of *Aedes aegypti* in Northeastern México. Journal of the American Mosquito Control Association. 2001;**17**:93-97

[33] Fávaro EA, Mondini A, Dibo MR, Barbosa AAC, Eiras AE, Chiavalloti-Neto FC. Assessment of entomological indicators of *Aedes aegypti* (L.) from adult and egg collections in São Paulo, Brazilian. Journal of Vector Ecology. 2008;**33**(1):8-16. DOI: 10.3376/1081-1710(2008)33[8:AOEIOA]2.0.CO;2

[34] Maciel-de-Freitas R, Peres RC, Alves F, Brandolini MB. Mosquito traps designed to capture *Aedes aegypti* (Diptera: Culicidae) females: Preliminary comparison of Adultrap, MosquiTRAP and backpack aspirator efficiency in a dengue-endemic area of Brazil. Memórias do Instituto Oswaldo Cruz. 2008;**103**(6):602-605. DOI: 10.1590/S0074-02762008000600016

[35] Codeço CT, Lima AW, Araújo SC, Lima JBP, Maciel-de-Freitas R, Honório NA, et al. Surveillance of *Aedes aegypti*: Comparison of house index with four alternative traps. PLoS Neglected Tropical Diseases. 2015;**9**(2):e0003475. DOI: 10.1371/journal.pntd.0003475

[36] DPO DM, Scherrer LR, Eiras AE. Dengue fever occurrence and vector detection by larval survey, ovitrap and MosquiTRAP: A space-time clusters analysis. PLoS One. 2012;**7**(7):e42125. DOI: 10.1371/journal.pone.0042125

[37] Regis LN, Acioli RV, Silveira JC, Melo-Santos MAV, Souza WV. Sustained reduction of the dengue vector population resulting from an integrated control strategy applied in two Brazilian cities. PLoS One. 2013;**8**(7):e67682. DOI: 10.1371/journal.pone.0067682

[38] Pepin KM, Leach CB, Marques-Toledo C, Laass KH, Paixao KS, Luis AD, et al. Utility of mosquito surveillance data for spatial prioritization of vector control against dengue viruses in three Brazilian cities. Parasites & Vectors. 2015;**8**:98. DOI: 10.1186/s13071-015-0659-y

[39] Ai-leen GT, Song RJ. The use of GIS in Ovitrap monitoring for dengue control in Singapore. Dengue Bulletin. 2000;**24**:110-116

[40] Regis L, Monteiro AM, Melo-Santos MAV, Silveira JC, Furtado AF, Acioli RV, et al. Developing new approaches for detecting and preventing *Aedes aegypti* population outbreaks: Basis for surveillance, alert and control system. Memórias do Instituto Oswaldo Cruz. 2008;**103**:50-59. DOI: 10.1590/S0074-02762008000100008

[41] Pepin KM, Marques-Toledo C, Scherer L, Morais MM, Ellis B, Eiras AE. Cost-effectiveness of novel system of mosquito surveillance and control, Brazil. Emerging Infectious Diseases. 2013;**19**(4):542-550. DOI: 10.3201/eid1904.120117

[42] Flacio E, Engeler L, Tonolla M, Lünthy P, Patocchi N. Strategies of a thirteen year surveillance programme on *Aedes albopictus* (*Stegomyia albopicta*) in southern Switzerland. Parasites & Vectors. 2015;**8**:208. DOI: 10.1186/s13071-015-0793-6

[43] Carrieri M, Albieri A, Angelini P, Baldacchini F, Venturelli C, Zeo SM, et al. Surveillance of the chikungunya vector *Aedes albopictus* (Skuse) in Emilia Romagna (Northern Italy): Organizational and technical aspects of a large scale monitoring system. Journal of Vector Ecology. 2011;**36**:108-118. DOI: 10.1111/j.1948-7134.2011.00147.x

[44] Arruda M, Vermulm R, Holland S. Technological Innovation in Brazil: The Industry in Search of Global Competitiveness. Sao Paulo: National Association of R&D of Innovative Companies; 2006

[45] Marques JS, Yigitcanlar T, Eduardo MDC. Incentivizing innovation: A review of the Brazilian Federal Innovation Support Programs. Asia Pacific Journal of Innovation and Entrepreneurship. 2015;**9**(1):31-56

[46] WHO-World Health Organization. Scientific Working Group. Report on Dengue. Geneva: WHO; 2006. 168 pp

[47] World Health Organization. Report of the Fourth Meeting of the Vector Control Advisory Group; 16-18 November 2015; 2016

[48] Sanavria A, Silva CB, Electo ÉH, Nogueira LCR, Thomé SMG, Angelo IC, et al. Intelligent monitoring of *Aedes aegypti* in a rural area of Rio de Janeiro State, Brazil. Revista do Instituto de Medicina Tropical de São Paulo. 2017;**59**:e51. DOI: 10.1590/s1678-9946201759051. Epub August 03

[49] Bangs MJ, Tan R, Listiyaningsih E, Kay BH, Porter KR. Detection of dengue viral RNA in *Aedes aegypti* (Diptera: Culicidae) exposed to sticky lures using reverse-transcriptase polymerase chain reaction. Journal of Medical Entomology. 2001;**38**(5):720-724

[50] dos Santos TP, Cruz OG, da Silva KAB, de Castro MG, de Brito AF, Maspero RC, et al. Dengue serotype circulation in natural populations of *Aedes aegypti*. Acta Tropica. 2017;**176**:140-143. DOI: 10.1016/j.actatropica.2017.07.014

[51] Blanco-Tuirán P, Camacho-Burgos E, Corrales-Aldana H, Ruiz-Contreras V. Detección molecular del virus dengue en mosquitos *Aedes aegypti* (Diptera: Culicidae) de la ciudad de Sincelejo, Colombia. Revista do Instituto de Medicina Tropical de São Paulo. 2015;**1**:1-7

[52] Ellis BR, Wilcox BA. The ecological dimensions of vector-borne disease research and control. Cadernos de Saúde Pública. 2009;**25**:S155-S167

[53] Sarkar S. Ecology. The Stanford Encyclopedia of Philosophy (Winter 2016 Edition). Zalta EN, editor. Available from: https://plato.stanford.edu/archives/win2016/entries/ecology/ [Accessed: December 6, 2017]

[54] Halstead SB. Dengue virus–mosquito interactions. Annual Review of Entomology. 2008;**53**:273-291

[55] Focks DA, Barrera R. Dengue transmission dynamics: Assessment and implications for control. In: Report of the Scientific Working Group Meeting on Dengue. Geneva: WHO; Oct. 2006. pp. 92-109

[56] Johansson MA, Dominici F, Glass GE. Local and global effects of climate on dengue transmission in Puerto Rico. PLoS Neglected Tropical Diseases. 2009;**3**(2):e382

[57] Gubler DJ. The global emergence/resurgence of arboviral diseases as

public health problems. Archives of Medical Research. 2002;**33**(4):330-342

[58] Watts DM, Burke DS, Harrison BA, Whitmire RE, Nisalak A. Effect of temperature on the vector efficiency of *Aedes aegypti* for dengue 2 virus. The American Journal of Tropical Medicine and Hygiene. 1987;**36**(1): 143-152

[59] Simões TC, Codeço CT, Nobre AA, Eiras AE. Modeling the non-stationary climate dependent temporal dynamics of *Aedes aegypti*. PLoS One. 2013;**8**(8):e64773

[60] Barsante LS, Cardoso RTN, Acebal JL, Moraes MM, Eiras AE. Relationship between rainfall and control effectiveness of the *Aedes aegypti* population through a non-linear dynamical model: Case of Lavras city, Brazil. In: Mondaini RP, editor. Biomat. Hackensack, New Jersey: World Scientific Publishing Co. Pte. Ltd; 2012, 2013. pp. 256-267

[61] Sedda L, Vilela APP, Aguiar ERGR Gaspar CHP, Gonçalves ANA, Olmo RP, Silva ATS, et al. The spatial and temporal scales of local dengue virus transmission in natural settings: A retrospective analysis. Parasites & Vectors. 2018;**11**:1-14

[62] Lana RM, Martins LR, Morais MM, Lima TFM, Carneiro TGSG, Stolerman LM, et al. Assessment of a trap based *Aedes aegypti* surveillance program using mathematical modeling. PLoS One. 2018;**13**:e0190673

[63] Chadee DD, Williams FL, Kitron UD. Impact of vector control on a dengue fever outbreak in Trinidad, West Indies, in 1998. Tropical Medicine & International Health. 2005;**10**(8):748-754

[64] Yang HM, Macoris ML, Galvani KC, Andrighetti MT, Wanderley DM. Assessing the effects of temperature on the population of *Aedes aegypti*, the vector of dengue. Epidemiology and Infection. 2009;**137**(8):1188-1202

[65] Beserra EB, Castro FP Jr, Santos JW, Santos TD, Fernandes CR. Biology and thermal exigency of *Aedes aegypti* (L.) (Diptera: Culicidae) from four bioclimatic localities of Paraiba. Neotropical Entomology. 2006;**35**(6):853-860

[66] Lambrechts L, Paaijmans KP, Fansiri T, Carrington LB, Kramer LD, Thomas MB, et al. Impact of daily temperature fluctuations on dengue virus transmission by *Aedes aegypti*. Proceedings of the National Academy of Sciences. 2011;**108**(18):7460-7465

[67] Hales S, De Wet N, Maindonald J, Woodward A. Potential effect of population and climate changes on global distribution of dengue fever: An empirical model. The Lancet. 2002;**360**(9336):830-834

[68] Canyon DV, Hii JL, Müller R. Adaptation of *Aedes aegypti* (Diptera: Culicidae) oviposition behavior in response to humidity and diet. Journal of Insect Physiology. 1999;**45**(10):959-964

[69] Brady OJ, Johansson MA, Guerra CA, Bhatt S, Golding N, Pigott DM, et al. Modelling adult *Aedes aegypti* and *Aedes albopictus* survival at different temperatures in laboratory and field settings. Parasites & Vectors. 2013;**6**(1):351

[70] Waldock J, Chandra NL, Lelieveld J, Proestos Y, Michael E, Christophides G, et al. The role of environmental variables on *Aedes albopictus* biology and chikungunya epidemiology. Pathogens and Global Health. 2013;**107**(5):224-241

[71] Moore CG, Cline BL, Ruiz-Tibén E, Lee D, Romney-Joseph H, Rivera-Correa E. *Aedes aegypti* in Puerto Rico: Environmental determinants of larval

abundance and relation to dengue virus transmission. The American Journal of Tropical Medicine and Hygiene. 1978;**27**(6):1225-1231

[72] Focks DA, Haile DG, Daniels E, Mount GA. Dynamic life table model for *Aedes aegypti* (Diptera: Culicidae): Analysis of the literature and model development. Journal of Medical Entomology. 1993;**30**(6):1003-1017

[73] Focks DA, Daniels E, Haile DG, Keesling JE. A simulation model of the epidemiology of urban dengue fever: Literature analysis, model development, preliminary validation, and samples of simulation results. The American Journal of Tropical Medicine and Hygiene. 1995;**53**(5):489-506

[74] Otero M, Solari HG, Schweigmann N. A stochastic population dynamics model for *Aedes aegypti*: Formulation and application to a city with temperate climate. Bulletin of Mathematical Biology. 2006;**68**(8):1945-1974

[75] Yang HM, Ferreira CP. Assessing the effects of vector control on dengue transmission. Applied Mathematics and Computation. 2008;**198**(1):401-413

[76] Pinho ST, Ferreira CP, Esteva L, Barreto FR, e Silva VM, Teixeira MG. Modelling the dynamics of dengue real epidemics. Philosophical Transactions. Series A, Mathematical, Physical, and Engineering Sciences. 2010;**368**(1933):5679-5693

[77] Yang HM, da Graca Macoris MD, Galvani KC, Andrighetti MT. Follow up estimation of *Aedes aegypti* entomological parameters and mathematical modellings. Bio Systems. 2011;**103**(3):360-371

[78] Aznar VR, Otero M, De Majo MS, Fischer S, Solari HG. Modeling the complex hatching and development of *Aedes aegypti* in temperate climates. Ecological Modelling. 2013;**253**:44-55

[79] MS - Ministério da Saúde. Diretrizes nacionais para prevenção e controle de epidemias de dengue, Secretaria de Vigilância em Saúde/Departamento de Vigilância Epidemiológica, Brasília; 2009. 160pp

[80] Suaya JA, Shepard DS, Siqueira JB, Martelli CT, Lum LC, Tan LH, et al. Cost of dengue cases in eight countries in the Americas and Asia: A prospective study. The American Journal of Tropical Medicine and Hygiene. 2009;**80**(5):846-855

[81] Alfaro-Murillo JA, Parpia AS, Fitzpatrick MC, Tamagnan JA, Medlock J, Ndeffo-Mbah ML, et al. A cost-effectiveness tool for informing policies on Zika virus control. PLoS Neglected Tropical Diseases. 2016;**10**(5):e0004743. DOI: 10.1371/journal.pntd.0004743

[82] Patterson J, Sammon M, Garg M. Dengue, Zika and Chikungunya: Emerging arboviruses in the new world. The Western Journal of Emergency Medicine. 2016;**17**(6):671

Chapter 8

Commercial Mosquito Repellents and Their Safety Concerns

Hanem Fathy Khater, Abdelfattah M. Selim, Galal A. Abouelella, Nour A. Abouelella, Kadarkarai Murugan, Nelissa P. Vaz and Marimuthu Govindarajan

Abstract

Mosquitoes are serious vectors of diseases threading millions of humans and animals worldwide, as malaria, filariasis, and important arboviruses like dengue, yellow fever, chikungunya, West Nile virus, and Zika viruses. The swift spread of arboviruses, parasites, and bacteria in conjunction with the development of resistance in the pathogens, parasites, and vectors represents a great challenge in modern parasitology and tropical medicine. Unfortunately, synthetic insecticides had led to some serious health and risk concerns. There are no vaccines or other specific treatments for arboviruses transmitted by mosquitoes. Accordingly, avoidance of mosquito bites remains the first line of defense. Insect repellents usually work by providing a vapor barrier deterring mosquitoes from coming into contact with the skin surface, and this chapter focused on assets and liabilities, mechanism of action, improving efficacy, safety, and future perspective of synthetic and natural repellents that could potentially prevent mosquito-host interactions, thereby playing an important role in reducing mosquito-borne diseases when used correctly and consistently.

Keywords: repellent plants, synthetic repellents, treated clothes, nanoparticles, microencapsulation

1. Introduction

Parasites since antiquity [1] are a serious threat for millions of humans and animals worldwide which bring about chronic debilitating, periodically disabling disease and are responsible for the overwhelming financial loss [2–6]. Mosquitoes (*Diptera*: *Culicidae*) [7, 8] are among them as they can act as vectors for serious parasites and pathogens, including malaria, filariasis, and important arboviruses, such as dengue, yellow fever, chikungunya, West Nile virus, and Zika viruses [9, 10]. Mosquito control and personal protection from mosquito bites are the most meaningful measures for controlling several life-threatening diseases transmitted exclusively by bites from bloodsucking mosquitoes. Repellents evolved, dates back to antiquity; the Pharaoh Sneferu, reigned from around 2613–2589 BCE and the founder of the fourth dynasty of Egypt, and Cleopatra VII, the last pharaoh of ancient Egypt, used bed nets as protection against mosquitoes; the ancient Egyptians used essential oils (EOs) for repelling insects, medicinal benefits, beauty care, and spiritual enhancement and in literally all aspects of their daily life [1]. Insect-repellent plants have been applied traditionally for thousands of years through different civilizations [11]. Such plants were used in various forms such as hanged bruised plants in houses, crude fumigants where plants were burnt to drive away mosquitoes, and oil formulations applied to the skin or clothes [12]. Smoke is undoubtedly the most extensively exploited means of repelling mosquitoes, typically by burning plants in rural tropics and by utilizing spiral-shaped incenses like Katori Senk—an archetypal icon of the humid Japanese summers [13].

Mosquitoes have been considered as a major obstacle to the tourism industry and socioeconomic development of developing countries particularly in the tropical and endemic regions [14]. Mosquito problems are ancient as old as the pyramids, and the presence of malaria in Egypt from circa 800 BCE onward has been confirmed using DNA-based methods, and antigens produced by *Plasmodium falciparum* leading to tertian fever in mummies from all periods were detected, and all mummies were suffering from malaria at the time of their death [1]. Herodotus noted down that the builders of the Egyptian pyramids (circa 2700–1700 BCE) were given large amounts of garlic almost certainly to protect them against malaria [1]. Despite recent considerable efforts to control vector-borne diseases, malaria alone produces 250 million cases per year and 800,000 deaths including 85% of children under 5 years [15]. Global warming has moved the mosquitoes on the way to some temperate and higher altitudes, affecting people who are vulnerable to such diseases [16]. Recently, malaria is a great problem in Africa, but it was well controlled in Egypt [1]. Ahead of the development and commercial success of synthetic insecticides in the mid-1930–1950s, botanical insecticides were the leading weapons for insect control. Synthetic insecticides are distinguished by their efficacy, speed of action, ease of use, and low cost. Therefore, they drove many natural control methods as botanicals, predators, and parasitoids to shadows [8, 17, 18]. Insecticidal treatment of house walls, in particular, could provide a very helpful reduction of mosquito incidence, but such measures need financial and organizational demand, but poor rural areas in endemic regions do not have sufficient resources for such costly protective measures. Because of health and environmental concerns [8, 17], there is an urgent need to identify new nonhazardous vector management strategies that replace harmful chemical insecticides and repellents. There are no vaccines or other specific treatments for arboviruses transmitted by mosquitoes; therefore, avoidance of mosquito bites remains the first line of defense [9, 18]. Hence, the use of the mosquito repellents (MRs) on exposed skin area is highly recommended.

Insect repellents usually work by providing a vapor barrier deterring mosquitoes from meeting the skin surface. Insect repellents had been used for thousands of years against biting arthropods. Several species of primates were observed anointing their pelage via rubbing millipedes and plants as *Citrus* spp., *Piper marginatum*, and *Clematis dioica*. Wedge-capped capuchins (*Cebus olivaceus*) were observed rubbing the millipede *Orthoporus dorsovittatus* onto their coat during the period of maximum mosquito activity [19]. Such millipede contains benzoquinones and insect-repellent chemicals, and it was hypothesized that the anointing behavior was intended to deter biting insects. Laboratory studies revealed a significant repellent effect of benzoquinones against *Aedes* (*Stegomyia*) *aegypti* (the yellow fever mosquito) and *Amblyomma americanum* (the lone star tick). Such anointing behavior to deter blood-feeding arthropods is also common among birds, and it could be genetically expressed as an "extended phenotype" as it has an obvious adaptive advantage. Evidence for this lies in the fact that benzoquinones applied to filter paper elicited anointing activity among captive-born capuchins [12]. The World Health Organization (WHO) also recommends repellents for protection against malaria as the resistance of *Plasmodium falciparum* to anti-malarial drugs such as chloroquine is increased. Most of the commercial MRs are prepared using non-biodegradable, synthetic chemicals like *N*,*N*-diethyl-3-methylbenzamide (DEET), dimethylphthalate (DMP), and allethrin which may lead to the environment and, hence, the unacceptable health risks in the case of their higher exposure. With an increasing concern for public safety, a renewed interest in the use of natural products of plant origin is desired because natural products are effective, environmentally friendly, biodegradable, inexpensive, and readily available [7, 8, 13, 17, 20]. Repellent application is a reliable mean of personal protection against annoyance and pathogenic infections not only for local people but also for travelers in disease risk areas, particularly in tropical countries; therefore, this chapter focused on assets and liabilities, safety, and future perspective of synthetic and natural MRs that could potentially prevent mosquito-host interactions, thereby playing an important role in reducing mosquito-borne diseases when used correctly and consistently.

2. Synthetic repellents

The history of synthetic repellents had been reviewed [12]; before World War II, MRs were primarily plant-based with the oil of citronella being the most widely used compound and the standard against which others were evaluated. At that time, the emergence of synthetic chemical repellents starts. There were only three principal repellents: dimethylphthalate discovered in 1929, Indalone® (butyl-3,3-dihydro-2,2-dimethyl-4-oxo-2*H*-pyran-6-carboxylate) patented in 1937, and Rutgers 612 (ethyl hexanediol), which became available in 1939. Later on and for military use, 6-2-2 of M-250 (a mixture of six parts DMP and two parts each Indalone® and Rutgers 612) was used [13]. The event of World War II was the primary switch on in the development of new repellent technologies because the Pacific and North African theaters posed significant disease threats to allied military personnel. Over 6000 chemicals had been tested from 1942 to 1947 in a variety of research institutions led to the identification of multiple successful repellent chemistries. Such great aim established several independent research projects that inevitably identified one of the most effective and widely used insect repellents to date, DEET. From then on, several compounds have been synthesized relying on previous research, which identified amide and imide compounds as highly successful contact repellents. Among these are picaridin, a piperidine carboxylate ester, and IR3535, which are currently considered DEET competitors in some repellency bioassays [21]. The chemical structures of some synthetic repellents are shown in **Figure 1**.

2.1 DEET

DEET (*N*,*N*-diethyl-3-methylbenzamide) is the standard and most effective broad-spectrum insect-repellent component with a long-lasting effect on mosquitoes, ticks, as well as biting flies, chiggers, and fleas. DEET was discovered as a mosquito repellent by the US Department of Agriculture and patented by the US Army in 1946. It was allowed for public use in 1957, and since then it has been a standard repellent for several insects and arthropods [14]. DEET is the most studied insect repellent and mainly used as a positive control to compare the efficacy of many repellent substances. DEET has a dose-dependent response: the higher the concentration, the longer the protection. DEET, 20–25%, is the conventional concentration used in commercial products. The shorter protection time depended on the mixture as well [14]. In fact, DEET plays a limited role on

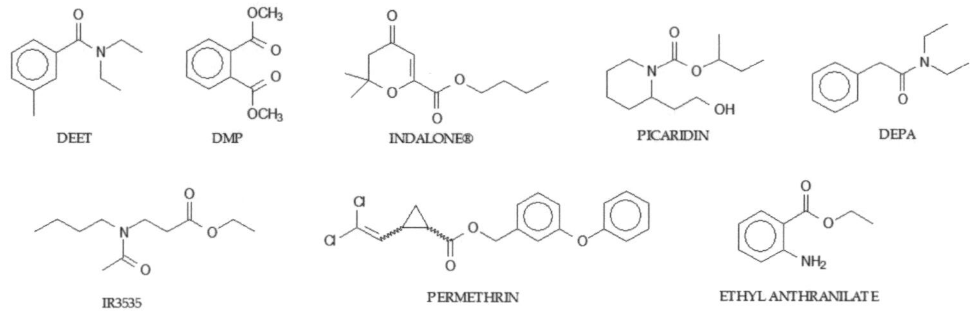

Figure 1.
Chemical structures of some synthetic repellents.

disease control in endemic regions because of its high cost, unpleasant odor, and inconvenience of the continuous application on the exposed skin at high concentrations [22, 23].

2.2 Permethrin

Permethrin is a pyrethroid insecticide derived from the plant *Chrysanthemum cinerariifolium*. It was registered in the US in 1979 as both repellent and insecticide. Recently, it is the most common insecticide available for use on fabrics such as clothing, bed nets, etc. for its exclusive role as a contact insecticide via neural toxicity and equally as an insect repellent [7, 8, 13, 17]. The protection offered against a broad range of bloodsucking arthropods with negligible safety concerns ranked permethrin-treated clothing an important arthropod protection technique especially when used in combination with other protection strategies as applying topical repellents [13].

2.3 Picaridin

Picaridin (1-piperidinecarboxylic acid 2-(2-hydroxyethyl)-1-methylpropylester) is a colorless, nearly odorless piperidine analog that was developed by Bayer in the 1980s through molecular modeling [12]. It is also known as KBR 3023, icaridin, hydroxyethyl isobutyl piperidine carboxylate, and *sec*-butyl-2-(2-hydroxyethyl)-piperidine-1-carboxylate. Its trade names include Bayrepel and Saltidin, among others. Picaridin was first marketed in Europe in the 1990s and later in the US in 2005 [24, 25]. The efficacy of picaridin is as good as DEET, and notably, 20% picaridin spray was found to protect against three main mosquito vectors, *Aedes*, *Anopheles*, and *Culex* for about 5 h with better efficacy than that of DEET. Therefore, repeated application is required every after 4–6 h [13]. In Australia, a formulation containing 19.2% picaridin provided similar protection as 20% DEET against *Verrallina lineata* [26]. The same formulation provided >95% protection against *Culex annulirostris* for 5 h but only 1-hour protection against *Anopheles* spp. [26]. Picaridin at concentrations of 2–13% *v/v* in 90% ethanol showed better protection against anophelines in Africa than comparable formulations containing DEET [27]. Field studies against mosquitoes in two locations in Australia indicated that a 9.3% formulation only provided 2-hour protection against *V. lineata* [26, 28]. It had been concluded that studies showed little significant difference between DEET and picaridin when applied at the same dosage, with a superior persistence for picaridin [29]. To maintain effectiveness than with the higher concentrations (>20%) of picaridin used in the field.

2.4 DEPA

N,N-diethyl-2-phenyl-acetamide (DEPA) is a repellent developed around the same time as DEET and repels a wide range of insects, but DEPA did not get its reputation. The repellency of DEPA has demonstrated almost similar to DEET against mosquito vectors as *Ae. aegypti*, *Ae. albopictus*, *An. stephensi*, and *C. quinquefasciatus* [13]. It has regained interest recently and could prove to be an important competitor to DEET especially in developing countries due to its low cost, $25.40 per kg compared to $48.40 per kg for DEET [30].

2.5 Insect repellent 3535

Learning from nature offered a molecule with an impressive performance in comparison to a natural and pure synthetic repellent solution called insect repellent 3535 (IR3535). Scientists got inspirations from nature for the development of the topical IR 3535 with the intention to create a molecule with optimized protection times and low toxicity. The naturally occurring amino acid β-alanine was used as a basic module, and the selected end groups were chosen to avoid toxicity and increase efficacy. IR 3535 was developed by Merck in 1970 and thus named as Merck IR3535; it has been available in Europe, but it was not available in the USA until 1999 [12]. IR3535 is used for humans and animals, as it is effective against mosquitoes, ticks, flies, fleas, and lice. Its chemical formula is $C_{11}H_{21}NO_3$, and its other names are ethyl-*N*-acetyl-*N*-butyl-β-alaninate, ethyl butylacetylaminopropionate (EBAAP), β-alanine, and *N*-acetyl-*N*-butyl-ethyl ester. The protection of IR 3535 may be comparable to DEET, but it requires frequent reapplication in every 6–8 h. IR3535 is found in products including Skin So Soft Bug Guard Plus Expedition (Avon, New York, NY) [31]. Although 20% IR 3535 provides complete protection against *Aedes* and *Culex* mosquitoes (up to 7–10 h), it offers lesser protection against *Anopheles* (about 3.8 h), which affects its application in malaria-endemic areas [13]. Several field studies were identified and indicated that IR 3535 is as effective as similarly, DEET in repelling mosquitoes of the *Aedes* and *Culex* genera but may be less effective than DEET in repelling anopheline mosquitoes; an uncontrolled field study of a controlled release formulation of IR 3535 reported that these formulations may provide complete protection against mosquito biting for 7.1–10.3 h [32].

2.6 Ethyl anthranilate

Ethyl anthranilate (EA) is a new member in the scope of entomology which drew a significant attention in repellent research in the recent years and is being considered as an improved alternative to DEET [13, 33]. It is a nontoxic, the US FDA approved volatile food additive. EA is novel and repellent against *Ae. aegypti*, *An. stephensi*, and *Cx. quinquefasciatus* as its ED_{50} values of EA were 0.96, 5.4, and 3.6% *w/v*, respectively, and CPTs of EA, 10% *w/v*, throughout the arm-in-cage method were 60, 60, and 30 min, respectively. Moreover, its spatial repellency was found to be extremely effective in repelling all the three tested species of mosquitoes. EA provided comparable results to standard repellent DEPA. As a result, the repellent activity of EA is promising for developing effective, safe, and eco-friendly alternative to the existing harmful repellents for personal protection against different mosquito species [34].

2.7 Comparative efficacy of synthetic repellents

The comparative efficacy of synthetic repellents had been summarized [14] as follows: *Aedes* species demonstrated an aggressive biting behavior and *Ae. Aegypti*, above all, proved to be tolerant to many repellent products. *Ae. albopictus* was easier to be repelled than *Ae. aegypti*. DEET is the most studied insect repellent; at higher concentrations, it presented superior efficacy against *Aedes* species, providing up to 10 h of protection. Although IR3535 and picaridin showed good repellency against this mosquito genus, their efficacy was on average inferior to that provided by DEET. Fewer studies have been conducted on the mosquito species *Anopheles* and *Culex*. The repellency profile against *Anopheles* species was similar for the four principal repellents of interest: DEET provided on average 5–11 h, IR 3535 4–10 h, picaridin 6–8 h, and *Citriodora* 1–12 h of protection, depending on study conditions and repellent concentration. *Culex* mosquitoes are easier to repel, and each repellent provided good protection against this species. DEET showed 5–14 h of protection and IR 3535 2–15 h, depending on product concentration, while the test proving the efficacy of picaridin and commercial products containing PMD was discontinued after 8 h of protection. To go over the main points, DEET remains probably the most efficient insect repellent against mosquitoes, effective against sensitive species as *Culex* as well as more repellent-tolerant species such as *Aedes* and *Anopheles*. Even though fewer studies have been conducted on these non-DEET compounds, picaridin and to some extent IR 3535 represent valid alternatives. Consequently, the choice of repellents could be adjusted somehow according to the profile of biting vectors at the travelers' destination.

3. Botanicals

Nature is an old unlimited source of inspiration for people [1, 11, 18, 35] as well as for scientific and technological innovations. Recently, global attention has been paid toward exploring the medicinal benefits of plant extracts [4, 11, 36, 37]. Repellents of natural origin are derived from members of the families as *Asteraceae*, *Cupressaceae*, *Labiatae*, *Lamiaceae*, *Lauraceae*, *Meliaceae*, *Myrtaceae*, *Piperaceae*, *Poaceae*, *Rutaceae*, *Umbelliferae*, and *Zingiberaceae*. They have been evaluated for repellency against various mosquito vectors, but few compounds have been found commercially. Increased curiosity in plant-based arthropod repellents was generated after the United States Environmental Protection Agency (US EPA) added a rule to the Federal Insecticide, Fungicide and Rodenticide Act (FIFRA) in 1986 exempting compounds considered to be minimum hazardous pesticides [30]. Increased interest has also been driven by the rapid registration process of plant-based repellents by US EPA, which are often registered in less than a year, while the conventional pesticides are registered in an average of 3 years [30]. The public considers botanicals as safer and suitable alternative repellents; most of them are produced and distributed locally and appear on the market for only a short time. Even though many studies have shown that almost all registered commercial products based on botanical active ingredients offer limited protection and require frequent reapplication than even a low concentration of DEET-based repellents, the growing demand for natural alternative repellents in the community illustrates further need to evaluate new botanical repellents critically for personal protection against mosquitoes and mosquito-borne illnesses [7, 8, 13, 17]. The repellent activity of EOs includes some metabolites, such as the monoterpenes α-pinene, cineole, eugenol, limonene, terpinolene, citronellol, citronellal, camphor, and thymol that are repellents against mosquitoes; the sesquiterpene, β-caryophyllene, is repellent against *A. aegypti*, and phytol, a linear diterpene alcohol, is repellent against *Anopheles gambia*. Most of the arthropod-repellent compounds are oxygenated, having the hydroxyl group linked to a primary, secondary, or aromatic carbon. In some metabolites having a hydroxyl group linked to a tertiary carbon, as linalool,

α-terpineol, and limonene, the repellent activity is suppressed against *A. gambiae*, suggesting the likelihood that the type of carbon where the hydroxyl substitution is there modulates repellency. Most insect repellents are volatile terpenoids such as terpinen-4-ol. Other terpenoids can act as attractants. More information is widely discussed [7, 38], and chemical structures of some natural repellent compounds are shown in **Figure 2**.

3.1 PMD and lemon-scented eucalyptus

Compound *p*-menthane-3,8-diol (PMD is derived from lemon-scented eucalyptus (*Eucalyptus citriodora*, *Myrtaceae*) leaves, and its importance as a repelling agent is increasing due to its good efficacy profile as well as its natural basis. PMD is a potent and commercially available repellent discovered in the 1960s via mass screening of plants for repellent activity, for instance, lemon eucalyptus and *Corymbia citriodora* (*Myrtaceae*) formerly known as *Eucalyptus maculata citriodora*. Lemon eucalyptus EO contains 85% citronellal and is already used in cosmetic industries due to its fresh smell. It was discovered when the waste distillate remaining after hydro-distillation of the EO was far more effective at repelling mosquitoes than the EO itself, and it provides very high protection from a broad range of insect vectors for several hours as well [7, 39]. The EO from *C. citriodora* also contains active constituents like citronella, citronellol, geraniol, isopulegol, and δ-pinene which play important roles in repelling both mosquitoes and ticks. Such compounds provide short-term repellency against mosquitoes, but PMD has a longer protection time than other plant-derived compounds because it is a monoterpene with low volatility than volatile monoterpenes found in most EOs and does not tend to evaporate rapidly after skin application [7, 8, 14].

There have been attempts to commercialize and market the insecticides/repellent products containing eucalyptus oil as such or based upon them. Crude eucalyptus oil was primarily registered as an insecticide and miticide in the USA in 1948, and 29 of such compounds have been registered in the USA until the year 2007 for use as natural insecticide/insect repellent/germicide. Only four products of them

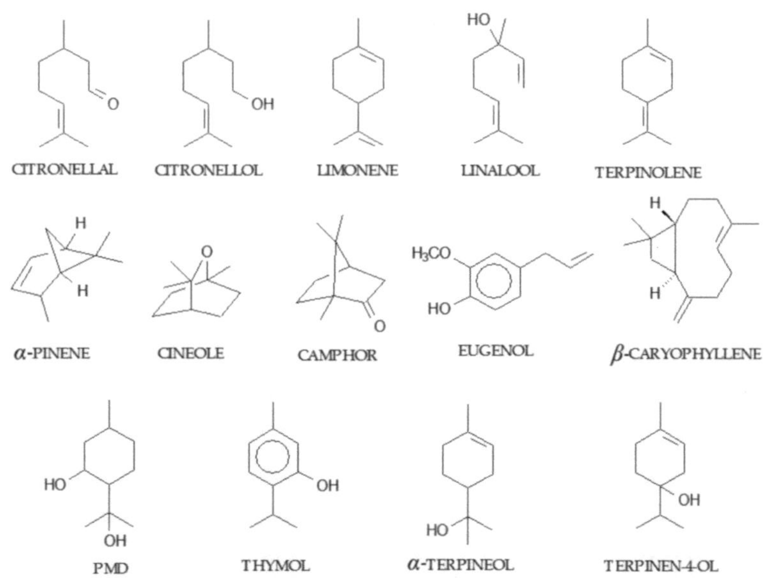

Figure 2.
Chemical structures of some natural repellent compounds found in botanical species.

have been active, whereas 25 have been canceled. These include Citriodiol, Repel essential insect repellent lotion (two variants), Repel essential insect repellent pump spray, and Repel insect repellent 30 by the United Industrial Corp., USA. Some eucalyptus-based products include the following: Quwenling is successfully marketed as an insect repellent in China and provides protection against anopheles mosquitoes parallel to DEET and has exchanged the widely used synthetic repellent dimethylphthalate; Quwenling contains a mixture of PMD, citronellol, and isopulegone. Mosiguard Natural contains 50% eucalyptus oil, Buzz Away is a commercially available product in China based on citronellal, and MyggA1 Natural is based on PMD from lemon eucalyptus and is shown to repel ticks. More details are widely discussed [40].

3.2 Citronella

The name "Citronella" is derived from the French word "citronelle" around 1858. It was extracted to be used in perfumery and used by the Indian Army to repel mosquitoes at the beginning of the twentieth century and was then registered for commercial use in the USA in 1948. Today, citronella (5–10%) is one of the most widely used natural repellents on the market; such concentrations are lower than most other commercial repellents, whereas higher concentrations can cause skin sensitivity. Among plant-derived substances, products containing Citriodiol showed the most effective repellent profile against mosquitoes. EOs and extracts belonging to plants in the *Citronella* genus (Poaceae) are commonly used as ingredients of plant-based mosquito repellents, mostly *Cymbopogon nardus* that is sold in Europe and North America in commercial preparations [39]. Citronella contains citronellal, citronellol, geraniol, citral, α-pinene, and limonene giving an effect similar to that of DEET, but the oils rapidly evaporate causing loss of efficacy and leaving the user unprotected. Among plant-derived substances, products containing Citriodiol showed the most effective repellent profile against mosquitoes. For travelers heading to disease-endemic areas, citronella-based repellents should not be recommended, but if efficacious alternatives are prohibitively expensive or not available, the use of citronella to prevent mosquito bites may provide important protection from disease vectors. Even though citronella-based repellents only give protection from host-seeking mosquitoes for a short time (2 h), formulations could prolong such time (please see the formulation section).

3.3 Neem and methyl jasmonate

The aromatic plants of the *Meliaceae* family which include neem, *Azadirachta indica*, *Carapa procera*, *Melia azedarach*, *Khaya senegalensis*, and *Trichilia emetica* contain substances of the limonoid group and insecticidal and repellent effects on insects [18]. Neem provided a protection of 98.2% for 8 h against *An. darlingi*. Regardless of being not approved by US EPA for use as a topical insect repellent, neem is widely advertised as a natural alternative to DEET, and it has been tested for repellency against a wide range of arthropods of medical and veterinary importance. MiteStop®, based on a neem seed extract, had a considerable repellent effect on bloodsucking mosquitoes, tabanids, ceratopogonids, simuliids, as well as licking flies [41]. Several field studies from India have shown the very high efficacy of neem-based preparations, contrasting with findings of intermediate repellency by other researchers. However, these contrasting results may be due to differing methodologies and the solvents used to carry the repellents.

Methyl jasmonate (MJ) is derived from the nonvolatile jasmonic acid and has the ultimate vapor pressure for a repellent (0.001 mmHg at 25°C) which is quite higher than DEET. It repels only *Cx. quinquefasciatus* but does not repel *Ae. aegypti*, *An. gambiae*, *Phlebotomus* flies, and *Glossina morsitans*, which restricts the application of MJ to *C. quinquefasciatus* mosquitoes only. On the other hand, MJ has been found to cause aversion in a number of ticks such as nymphal *I. ricinis* and *Hyalomma marginatum rufipes* Koch, etc. [30].

3.4 Essential oils

EOs are used against insects [20, 42–50] throughout the globe. EOs are distilled from members of the *Lamiaceae* (mint family), *Poaceae* (aromatic grasses), and *Pinaceae* (pine and cedar family). EOs could be used for farm animal protection against nuisance flies and lice [47]. Almost all of the botanical repellents are also used for food flavoring or in the perfume industry, indicating that they are safer than DEET. The most effective oils include thyme, geraniol, peppermint, cedar, patchouli, and clove that have been found to repel malaria, filarial, and yellow fever vectors for a period of 60–180 mins. Most of these EOs are highly volatile, and this contributes to their poor longevity as mosquito repellents. As a result, repellents containing only EOs in the absence of an active ingredient such as DEET should not be recommended as repellents for use in disease-endemic areas, whereas those containing high levels of EOs could cause skin irritation, especially in the presence of sunlight [39]. Although EOs effectively repel mosquitoes as irritants, repellents, antifeedants, or maskants, unfortunately, relatively few have been commercialized, despite being widely used in candles and as topical insect repellents. Botanical, herbal, or natural-based repellents include one or several plant EOs. These oils are considered safe by the EPA at low concentrations but provide a limited duration of protection against mosquitoes (<3 h). Citronella (discussed previously) is the principal and sometimes only active ingredient in many plant-based insect repellents [7]. Eucalyptus oil is used as an antifeedant mainly against biting insects as eucalyptus-based products used on humans as insect repellent can give protection from biting insects up to 8 h depending upon the concentration of the essential oil. Such repellent activity could be extended up to 8 days when eucalyptus EOs are applied on the clothes. Eucalyptus oil (30%) can prevent mosquito bite for 2 h; however, the oil must have at least 70% cineole content [40]. On the other hand, *E. citriodora* EO alone showed an insufficient protection against the three main mosquito species [14].

4. Safety of repellents

4.1 Safety of synthetic repellents

Insect repellents containing DEET are broadly used among populations. DEET should be used with caution as it may damage spandex, rayon, acetate, and pigmented leather and it could dissolve plastic and vinyl (e.g., eyeglass frames). Moreover, DEET damages synthetic fabrics and painted and varnished surfaces, precluding its use in bed nets and in many urban settings [51]. Being the gold standard of repellents, the safety profile of DEET is largely studied. There is an estimated 15 million people in the UK, 78 million people in the USA, and 200 million people globally that use DEET each year safely when it is applied to the skin at the correct dose indicated at the commercial preparation (in the case of it not being swallowed or rubbed into the mucous membranes). DEET has been used since 1946 with a tiny number of reported adverse effects, many of which had a history of excessive or inappropriate use of repellent. Its toxicology has been more closely scrutinized than any other repellent, and it has been deemed safe for human use, including its use on children, pregnant women, and lactating women [39]. Even though insect repellents containing DEET are safe, some side effects have been described, mainly after inappropriate use such as dermatitis, allergic reactions, neurologic and cardiovascular side effects, as well as encephalopathy in children. In addition, there are a small number of reports of systemic toxicity in adults following dermal application. The safety profile in the second and third trimester of pregnancy has been well known through inspection of very low placental cord concentrations after maternal application of DEET, but animal models do not indicate any teratogenic effects. DEET also blocks mammalian sodium and potassium ion channels contributing to the numbness of lip following the application of DEET [13]. Approval for use in young children is a controversial issue between countries, with some recommending lower concentrations, whereas others suggesting that higher strengths can be used. However, the causation between the few reported cases of encephalopathy in children and the topical use of DEET cannot be supported by a good evidence base [14, 39].

When permethrin is impregnated appropriately in cloths and nets, toxicity fearfulness is minimal [52]. Although synthetic pyrethroids are utilized worldwide as active ingredients in MRs [15] due to their relatively low toxicity to mammals [53], inappropriate application at high doses initiates neurotoxic effects such as tremors, loss of coordination, hyperactivity, paralysis, and an increase in body temperature. Other side effects include skin and eye irritation, reproductive effects, mutagenicity, alterations in the immune system, etc. [13]. Recent studies also showed that some pyrethroids are listed as endocrine disruptors and possible carcinogens [53] and pyrethroids might cause behavioral and developmental neurotoxicity, with special concern revolving around infants and children, due to their potential exposure during a sensitive neurodevelopmental stage [54]. More evidence in the recent years indicates that pyrethroid insecticides can reduce sperm count and motility, cause deformity of the sperm head, increase the count of abnormal sperm, damage sperm DNA, induce its aneuploidy rate, affect sex hormone levels, and produce reproductive toxicity [55]. Moreover, an elevated concentration of transfluthrin in the gaseous phase during the indoor application of an electric vaporizer was detected, but they found inhalation risk of airborne transfluthrin was low. The exposure levels and potential risk of pyrethroids during the applications of other types of commonly used MRs remain unknown [53]. On the other hand, long-term exposure to pyrethroid-based MRs in indoor environments causes chronic neurotoxicity, for example, dysfunction of blood-brain barrier permeability, oxidative damage to the brain, [56] and cholinergic dysfunction which cause learning and memory deficiencies [57]. Even though ventilation through natural air exchange and conditioner dissipate of airborne pollutants, residues persisting in the air and/or on indoor surfaces could potentially cause continuous exposure to the residents.

US EPA-OPP's Biochemical Classification Committee classified IR 3535 as a biochemical in 1997, because it is functionally identical to naturally occurring beta-alanine in that both repel insects, the basic molecular structure is identical, the end groups are not likely to contribute to toxicity, and it acts to control the target pest via a nontoxic mode of action [58]. No reported toxicity has been made so far against IR 3535, and it induces less irritation to mucous membranes and exhibits safer oral and dermal toxicity than DEET which makes it an attractive alternative to DEET in disease-inflicted endemic regions [13]. The ester structure of the propionate grants essential advantages because of a short metabolic degradation and quick excretion as a simple water-soluble acid [58]. Picaridin has the advantage of being odorless and non-sticky or greasy. Moreover, unlike DEET, picaridin does not damage plastics and synthetics. In some studies, picaridin induces no adverse toxic reactions in animal studies but exhibits low toxicity and less dermatologic and olfactory irritant in other studies. Consequently, picaridin's comparable efficacy to DEET and its suitability of application and favorable toxicity profile ranked it as an attractive option and unquestionably an acceptable alternative for protection against mosquitoes and other hematophagous arthropods to control the menace of vector-borne diseases in endemic areas [13]. DEPA does not show cytotoxicity or mutagenicity [59], thereby increasing its suitability in direct skin application. It also exhibits moderate oral toxicity (mouse oral LD_{50} 900 mg/kg) and low to moderate dermal toxicity (rabbit and female mouse LD_{50} of 3500 and 2200 mg/kg, respectively) [60]. Acute and subacute inhalation toxicity studies of DEPA have also been reported [61] which indicate its applicability as aerosol formulations. Indalone was an early synthetic repellent effective against both mosquitoes and ticks. It was even more effective than DEET; however, its chronic exposure induced kidney and liver damage in rodents which restricted its application [13]. EA is approved by the US FDA, WHO and European Food Safety Authority (EFSA) [62, 63]. Furthermore, EA has been listed in the "generally recognized as safe" [64] list by the Flavour and Extract Manufacturers Association (FEMA) [65]. EA does not damage synthetic fabrics, plastics, and painted and varnished surfaces which further widen the utility of EA in bed nets, cloths, and different surfaces in the endemic settings [14, 66].

4.2 Safety of plant-based repellents

Because many conventional pesticide products fall into disfavor with the public, botanical-based pesticides should become an increasingly popular choice as repellents. There is a perception that natural products are safer for skin application and for the environment, just because they are natural and used for a long time compared to synthetic non-biodegradable products [14]. In contrast to DEET, some natural repellents are safer than others, and plant-based repellents do not have this strictly tested safety evidence, and many botanical repellents have compounds that need to be used with caution [39]. PMD has no or very little toxicity to the environment and poses no risks to humans and animals. PMD has been developed and registered for use against public health pests and is available as a spray and lotion. Not much is known about the toxicity of eucalyptus oils; however, they have been categorized as GRAS by the US EPA. Further, the oral and acute LD_{50} of eucalyptus oil and cineole to rat is 4440 mg/kg body weight (BW) and 2480 mg/kg BW, respectively, making it much less toxic than pyrethrins (LD_{50} values 350–500 mg/kg BW; US EPA, 1993) and even technical grade pyrethrum (LD_{50} value 1500 mg/kg BW) [40]. PMD is an important component of commercial repellents in the US and registered by US EPA and Canadian Pest Management Regulatory Agency in 2000 and 2002, respectively [13]. In contrary, lemon eucalyptus EO does not have US EPA registration for use as an insect repellent. PMD is the only plant-based repellent that has been advocated for use in disease-endemic areas by the Centers for Disease Control (CDC), due to its proven clinical efficacy to prevent malaria, and is considered to pose no risk to human health [39]. In 2005, the US Centers for Disease Control and Prevention made use of its influence by endorsing products containing "oil of lemon eucalyptus" (PMD), along with picaridin and DEET as the most effective repellents of mosquito vectors carrying the West Nile virus [67]. PMD provides excellent safety profile with minimal toxicity. In studies using laboratory animals, PMD demonstrated no adverse effects apart from eye irritation. It is safe for both children and adults as the toxicity of PMD is very low. However, the label indicates it should not be used on children under the age of 3 [7].

The safety of neem is extensively reviewed; azadirachtin is nontoxic to mammals and did not show chronic toxicity. Even at high concentrations, neem products were neither mutagenic nor carcinogenic, and they did not produce any skin irritations or organic alterations in mice and rats. On the other hand, reversible reproduction disturbances could occur due to the daily feeding of aqueous leaf extract for 6 and 9 weeks led to infertility of rats at 66.7 and 100%, respectively. Using unprocessed and aqueous neem-based products should be encouraged if applied with care. The pure compound azadirachtin, the unprocessed materials, the aqueous extracts, and the seed oil are safe to use even as insecticides to protect stored food for human consumption, whereas nonaqueous extracts turn out to be relatively toxic [8]. From the ecological and environmental standpoint, azadirachtin is safe and nontoxic to fish, natural enemies, pollinators, birds, and other wildlife. Azadirachtin is classified by the US EPA as class IV (practically nontoxic) [7, 8, 17] as azadirachtin breaks down within 50–100 h in water and is degraded by sunlight as the half-life of azadirachtin is only 1 day, leaving no residues. Safety and advantages of EOs are widely discussed [7, 8, 17, 39]. There is a popular belief that EOs are benign and harmless to the user. Honestly, increasing the concentration of plant EOs as repellents could increase efficacy, but high concentrations may also cause contact dermatitis. Some of the purified terpenoid ingredients of EOs are moderately toxic to mammals. Because of their volatility, EOs have limited persistence under field conditions. With few exceptions, the oils themselves or products based on them are mostly nontoxic to mammals, birds, and fish. Many of the commercial products that include EOs (EOs) are on the *"generally recognized as safe"_* [64] list fully approved by the US FDA and EPA for food and beverage consumption. Moreover, EOs are usually devoid of long-term genotoxic risks, and some of them show a very clear antimutagenic capacity which could be linked to an anticarcinogenic activity. The prooxidant activity of EOs or some of their constituents, like that of some polyphenols, is capable of reducing local tumor volume or tumor cell proliferation by apoptotic and/or necrotic effects. Due to the capacity of EOs to interfere with mitochondrial functions, they may add prooxidant effects and thus become genuine antitumor agents. The cytotoxic capacity of the essential oils, based on a prooxidant activity, can make them outstanding antiseptic and antimicrobial agents for personal uses, that is, for purifying air, personal hygiene, or even internal use via oral consumption and for insecticidal use for the preservation of crops or food stocks. Some EOs acquired through diet are actually beneficial to human health [68, 69]. Eugenol is an eye and skin irritant and has been shown to be mutagenic and tumorigenic. Citronellol and 2-phenylethanol are skin irritants, and 2-phenylethanol is an eye irritant, mutagen, and tumorigenic; they also affect the reproductive and central nervous systems [30]. Hence, it is advised that EOs with toxic profile should be used for treating clothing rather than direct application to individual's skin [13]. Although EOs are exempt from registration through the US EPA, they can be irritating to the skin, and their repellent effect is variable, dependent on formulation and concentration. The previously mentioned safety and advantages designate that EOs could find their way from the traditional into the modern medical, insecticidal, and repellent domain.

5. Conclusions and challenges for future research

Several diseases transmitted by mosquitoes cause high losses of human and animal lives every year. DEET is considered as a "gold standard" to which other candidate repellents are compared; therefore, DEET is the most ever-present active ingredient used in commercially available repellents, with noteworthy protection against mosquitoes and other biting insects. Unfortunately, the widespread use and effectiveness of commercial formulations containing DEET and other synthetic substances could lead to resistance [70, 71]. Some health and environmental concerns lead to the search for natural alternative repellents. The use of repellent plants has been used since antiquity [1], and it is the only effective protection available for the poor people against vectors and their associated diseases [71]. Ethnobotanical experience is passed on orally from one generation to another, but it needs to be preserved in a written form and utilized as a rich source of botanicals in repellent bioassays. Then again, the growing demand for natural repellents points up the further necessity to evaluate new plant-based products critically for personal protection against mosquitoes and mosquito-borne diseases [7, 8, 17, 18]. Regarding environmental and health concerns, plant-based repellents are better than synthetic molecules. Even though many promising plant repellents are available, their use is still limited; therefore, advance understanding of the chemical ecology of pests and the mode of repellency would be helpful for identifying competitor semiochemicals that could be incorporated into attractant or repellent formulations. There are numerous commercially available formulations enhancing the longevity of repellent, by controlling the rate of delivery and the rate of evaporation. Such formulations are very useful to people living in the endemic areas in the form of sprays, creams, lotions, aerosols, oils, evaporators, patch, canister, protective clothing, insecticide-treated clothing, and insecticide-treated bed nets [7, 8, 17]. The potential uses and benefits of microencapsulation and nanotechnology are enormous including enhancement involving nanocapsules for pest management and nanosensors for pest detection [7, 8]. Nanoparticles are effectively used to control larvae [72–76] and to repel adults of mosquitoes [77, 78].

Polymer-based formulations allow entrapping active ingredients and provide release control. Encapsulation into polymeric micro/nanocapsules, cyclodextrins, polymeric micelles, or hydrogels constitutes an approach to modify physicochemical properties of encapsulated molecules. Such techniques, applied in topical formulations, fabric modification for personal protection, or food packaging, have been proven to be more effective in increasing repellency time and also in reducing drug dermal absorption, improving safety profiles of these products. In this work, the main synthetic and natural insect repellents are described as well as their polymeric carrier systems and their potential applications [79]. Encapsulated EO nanoemulsion is prepared to create stable droplets to increase the retention of the oil and slow down release. The release rate correlates well to the protection time so that a decrease in release rate can prolong mosquito protection time. Microencapsulation is another way to slowly release the active ingredients of repellents. In laboratory conditions, the microencapsulated formulations of the EOs showed no significant difference with regard to the duration of repellent effect compared to the microencapsulated DEET used at the highest concentration (20%). It exhibited >98% repellent effect for the duration of 4 h, whereas, in the field conditions, these formulations demonstrated the comparable repellent effect (100% for a duration of 3 h) to Citriodiol®-based repellent (Mosiguard®). In both test conditions, the microencapsulated formulations of the EOs presented longer duration of 100% repellent effect (between 1 and 2 h) than non-encapsulated formulations [80]. Microencapsulation reduces membrane permeation of CO while maintaining a constant supply of the citronella oil [81]. Moreover, using gelatin Arabic gum microcapsules also prolonged the effect of natural repellents. In addition, the functionalization of titanium dioxide nanoparticles on the surface of polymeric microcapsules was investigated as a mean to control the release of encapsulated citronella through solar radiation. The results showed that functionalizing the microcapsules with nanoparticles on their surface and then exposing them to

	Repellent composition	Dose	Study variety	Mosquito spp.	Mean CPT	Protection		Reference
						%	Time interval	
Bio Skincare®	Natural oil of jojoba, rapeseed, coconut, and vit. E	1.2 g/arm	Arm-in-cage	*An. arabiensis*		100 52	3–4 h 6 h	[85]
BioUD® spray	7.75% 2-undecanone	1 ml/600 cm^2	Arm-in-cage	*Ae. aegypti*		96.1 86.7 81.7 79.5 70.1 68.2	1 h 2 h 3 h 4 h 5 h 6 h	[86]
				Ae. albopictus		94.5 98.3 93.1 79.4 87.4 76.3	1 h 2 h 3 h 4 h 5 h 6 h	
	7.75% 2-undecanone	1 ml/600 cm^2	Field trial in North Carolina (USA)	*Ae. atlanticus/tormentor* (23.3%) *Psorophora ferox* (54.7%)		98.4 94.2 92.2 79	3 h 4 h 5 h 6 h	
			Field trial in Canada	*Ae. vexans* (32%) *Ae. euedes* (29.3%) *Ae. stimulans* (15.3%)		95.5 95.6	4 h 6 h	
Bite Blocker® lotion	Glycerin, lecithin, vanillin, oils of coconut, geranium, and soybean (2%)	1 ml/650 cm^2	Arm-in-cage	*Ae. albopictus* *Cx. nigripalus*	5.5 h 8.3 h			[87]
Bite Blocker Xtreme®	3% soybean oil 6% geranium oil 8% castor oil		Field trial in Canada	*Ae. vexans* (32%) *Ae. euedes* (29.3%) *Ae. stimulans* (15.3%)		93.9 53.7	4 h 6 h	[86]
Buzz Off Insect Repellent®	Natural plant extract	1 g/forearm	Arm-in-cage	*Ae. aegypti* *Ae. vigilax* *Cx. Annulirostris* *Cx. quinquefasciatus*	0 min 0 min 160 min 50 min			[88]
Baygon®	Oils of canola, eucalyptus, peppermint, rosemary, and sweet birch	1 ml/650 cm^2	Arm-in-cage	*Ae. albopictus* *Cx. nigripalus*	0.2 h 4.7 h			[87]

	Repellent composition	Dose	Study variety	Mosquito spp.	Mean CPT	Protection		Reference
						%	Time interval	
Citronella candles	3% citronella		Field trial in Canada	*Aedes* spp.		42.3		[89]
Citronella incense	5% citronella		Field trial in Canada	*Aedes* spp.		24.2		[89]
GonE!®	*Aloe vera*, camphor, menthol, oils of eucalyptus, lavender, rosemary, sage, and soybean	1 ml/650 cm^2		*Ae. albopictus* *Cx. nigripalus*	0.0 h 2.8 h			[87]
Green Ban for People®	Citronella 10%, peppermint oil 2%		Arm-in-cage	*Ae. aegypti*	14 min			[90]
Herbal Armor®	Citronella 12%, peppermint oil 2.5%, cedar oil 2%, lemongrass oil 1%, geranium oil 0.055		Arm-in-cage	*Ae. aegypti*	18.9 min			[90]
Kor Yor 15 DEET lotion®	DEET 24%, dimethylphthalate 24%	0.1 ml/30 cm^2	Arm-in-cage	*Ae. aegypti*	3 h			[91]
	DEET 24%, dimethylphthalate 24%	0.1 ml/30 cm^2	Arm-in-cage	*Ae. aegypti*	3 h			[92]
MeiMei® cream	Citronella and geranium oils		Indoor test	*Ae. aegypti*		97 97 85 44 27	30 min 50 min 70 min 90 min 120 min	[93]
	Citronella and geranium oils		Field trial in South Korea	*Aedes* (7.8%) *Armigeres* (5.9%) *Anopheles* (42.2%) *Culex* (44.1%)		90 57 56 34	30 min 90 min 150 min 210 min	[94]
Mistine censor®	IR 3535 12%, rosemary, lavender, and eucalyptus	0.1 ml/30 cm^2	Arm-in-cage	*Ae. aegypti*	1 h			[91]
	IR 3535 12%, rosemary, lavender, and eucalyptus	0.1 ml/30 cm^2	Arm-in-cage	*Ae. aegypti*	1 h			[92]
Mospel®	Clove oil 10% Makaen oil 10%	1 g/600 cm^2	Arm-in-cage	*An. stephensi*	4–5 h			[95]
		1 g/lower leg	Walk-in exposure room test		7–8 h			

	Repellent composition	Dose	Study variety	Mosquito spp.	Mean CPT	Protection		Reference
						%	Time interval	
MosquitoSafe®	Geraniol 25%, mineral oil 74%, aloe vera 1%	1 ml/550 cm^2	Arm-in-cage	*Ae. albopictus*	2.8 h			[87]
Neem Aura®	Aloe vera, extract of barberry, chamomile, goldenseal, myrrh, neem, and thyme; oil of anise, cedarwood, citronella, coconut, lavender, lemongrass, neem, orange, rhodium wood	1 ml/550 cm^2	Arm-in-cage	*Ae. albopictus* *Cx. nigripalus*	0.2 h 4.2 h			[87]
Odomos® cream	Advanced Odomos (12% N,N-diethylbenzamide)	8 mg/cm^2	Arm-in-cage (Duration of the test: 4 h)	*Cx. nigripalus*	3.8 h			[96]
		10 mg/cm^2			>4 h	100		
		10 mg/cm^2		*Ae. aegypti*	4 h	96.5		
		12 mg/cm^2			>4 h	100		
	Advanced odomos	10 mg/cm^2	Field trial in India Duration of the test: 11 h	*An. culicifacies* *An. stephensi* *An. annularis* *An. subpictus*	11 h	100		
		10 mg/cm^2		*Cx. quinquefasciatus*	9 h	98.8		
		10 mg/cm^2		*Ae. aegypti*	6.2 h	92.5		
Raid Dual Action and Raid Shield	transfluthrin-based spatial repellent products		Laboratory (wind tunnel) and	*Aedes aegypti*		95 and 74		[97]
			semi-field (outdoor enclosure) in Florida			88 and 66		

	Repellent composition	Dose	Study variety	Mosquito spp.	Mean CPT	Protection		Reference
						%	Time interval	
Repel Care®	Turmeric oil 5% *E. citriodora* 4.5%	2 ml/750 cm^2	Field trial in Thailand (duration of the test: 9 h)	*Ae. aegypti* (1.2%) *Others* (<1%) *Cx. vishnui* (77.1%) *Cx. quinquefasciatus* (13.8%) *Cx. gelidus* (3.4%) *Cx. tritaeniorhynchus* (1.6%)		100		
			Duration of the test: 8 h	*Ae. albopictus* (99.9%) *Ar. subalbatus* (0.01%)		100 96.9 92.4 91.8		
	Turmeric oil 5% *E. citriodora* 4.5%	0.1 ml/30 cm^2	Arm-in-cage	*Ae. aegypti*	1 h			[92]
Sketolene® lotion	DEET, *E. citriodora* oil 15%	0.1 ml/30 cm^2	Arm-in-cage	*Ae. aegypti*	3 h			[92]
Soffell® (citronella oil)	DEET 13%, citronella oil	0.1 ml/30 cm^2	Arm-in-cage	*Ae. aegypti*	4 h		[92]	
Soffell® (floral fragrance)	DEET 13%, geranium				4 h			
Soffell® (fresh fragrance)	DEET 13%, orange				4 h			
Soffell® lotion	DEET, *E. citriodora* oil 15%	0.1 ml/30 cm^2	Field trial in Thailand (duration of the test: 120 min)	*Ae. gardnerii* *Ae. lineatopennis* *An. barbirostris* *Cx. Tritaeniorhynchus* *Cx. gelidus*		100	(120 min)	[91]

	Repellent composition	Dose	Study variety	Mosquito spp.	Mean CPT	Protection		Reference
						%	Time interval	
Sumione®	Metofluthrin-treated emanators	900-cm² paper fan emanators impregnated with 160 mg metofluthrin	Field trials in PA, USA	*Aedes canadensis*		85–100		[98]
		4000-cm² paper strip emanators impregnated with 200 mg metofluthrin		Laboratory-reared *Aedes aegypti*		89–91		
		Metofluthrin-impregnated paper strip emanator	In Florida	*Ochlerotatus* spp.		91–95		
		Metofluthrin-impregnated paper strip emanator	In Washington State	*Aedes vexans*		95–97		
SunSwat®	Oils of bay, cedarwood, citronella, goldenseal, juniper, lavender, lemon peel, patchouli, pennyroyal, tansy, tea tree, and vetiver	1 ml/650 cm²	Arm-in-cage	*Ae. albopictus* *Cx. nigripalus*	0.2 h 4.2 h			[87]
Tipskin®	Bergamot oil, citronella oil, camphor oil, and vanillin	0.1 ml/30 cm²	Arm-in-cage	*Ae. aegypti*	0 h			[91]
	Bergamot oil, citronella oil, camphor oil, and vanillin	0.1 ml/30 cm²	Arm-in-cage	*Ae. aegypti*	0.5 h			[92]
OFF! Clip-On®	Metofluthrin		Field study in USA	*Ae. albopictus* and *Ae. taeniorhynchus*	3 h	70 and 79		[99]
				Anopheles quadrimaculatus, *Culex erraticus*, and *Psorophora columbiae*		Up to 84		[100]
Mosquito Cognito®	Linalool			*Anopheles quadrimaculatus*, *Culex erraticus*, and *Psorophora columbiae*		Up to 84		[100]
No-Pest Strip®	Dichlorvos							[100]
Thermacell®	d-*cis*/*trans* allethrin							[100]

Table 1.
Commercial mosquito-repellent products.

ultraviolet radiation effectively increased the output of citronella into the air for repelling the mosquitoes without human intervention, as the sunlight works as a release activator [82].

It is recommended to use US EPA-registered insect repellents including one of the active ingredients: DEET, Picaridin, IR3535, Oil of lemon eucalyptus (OLE), Para-menthane-diol (PMD), and 2-undecanone. Synthetic MRs are applied for years but induced some safety and environmental concerns; as a result, the advancement in the development of repellents from the botanical origin is encouraged. But some obstacles are hindering botanical repellents which as the source availability, standardization, commercialization, and analyses in order to certify the efficacy and safety [7]. Commercially available repellents are provided in **Table 1**. For saving time and efforts, a high-throughput chemical informatics screen via a structure-activity approach, molecular-based chemical prospecting [83], as well as computer-aided molecular modeling [84] would accelerate the exploration of new environmentally safe and cost-effective novel repellents which activated the same chemosensory pathways as DEET at a fairly shorter time and lower costs [13]. The selection of various repellents could be tailored along with the profile of safety concerns and biting vectors at the travelers' and military destinations by reducing annoyance and the incidence of illness. The use of these technologies to enhance the performance of natural repellents may revolutionize the repellent market and make EOs a more viable option for use in long-lasting repellents. Green technologies and cash cropping of repellent plants afford a vital source of income for small-scale farmers and producers in developing countries and raise the national economy. Moreover, in some developing countries where tourism is a chief source of national income, the use of repellents would increase the pleasure and comfort of tourists. Finally, much faster work needs to be done to discover new and safe repellents for personal protection from mosquitoes.

Author details

Hanem Fathy Khater[1*], Abdelfattah M. Selim[2], Galal A. Abouelella[3], Nour A. Abouelella[3], Kadarkarai Murugan[4], Nelissa P. Vaz[5] and Marimuthu Govindarajan[6]

1 Department of Parasitology, Faculty of Veterinary Medicine, Benha University, Toukh, Egypt

2 Department of Infectious Disease, Faculty of Veterinary Medicine, Benha University, Toukh, Egypt

3 Faculty of Pharmacy, British University of Egypt, Egypt

4 Division of Entomology, Department of Zoology, School of Life Sciences, Bharathiar University, Coimbatore, Tamil Nadu, India

5 Exact Sciences Sector—Department of Chemistry, Federal University of Paraná (UFPR), Curitiba, Paraná, Brazil

6 Unit of Vector Control, Phytochemistry and Nanotechnology, Department of Zoology, Annamalai University, Annamalainagar, Tamil Nadu, India

*Address all correspondence to: hanemkhater@gmail.com; hanem.salem@fvtm.bu.edu.eg

References

[1] Khater HF. Introductory chapter: Back to the future-solutions for parasitic problems as old as the pyramids. In: Natural Remedies in the Fight Against Parasites. Rijeka, Croatia: InTech; 2017

[2] Khalifa NO, Khater HF, Nassief MZ. Genetic fingerprint of unilocular hydatidosis in Egyptian camels and humans using nested PCR. Pakistan Veterinary Journal. 2014;**34**(4):522-526

[3] Ali A, Seddiek SA, Khater H. Effect of butyrate, clopidol and their combination on the performance of broilers infected with *Eimeria maxima*. British Poultry Science. 2014;**55**(4): 474-482

[4] Seddiek SA et al. The antitrichomonal efficacy of garlic and metronidazole against *Trichomonas gallinae* infecting domestic pigeons. Parasitology Research. 2014;**113**(4): 1319-1329

[5] Khater H, Khalifa N, Barakat A. Serological and molecular studies of ovine and human toxoplasmosis with a trial of treatment of infected ewe. Scientific Journal of Veterinary Advances. 2013;**2**:157-168

[6] El-Madawy R, Khalifa N, Khater H. Detection of cryptosporidial infection among Egyptian stray dogs by using *Cryptosporidium parvum* outer wall protein gene. Bulgarian Journal of Veterinary Medicine. 2010;**13**:104-110

[7] Khater H. Bioactivity of essential oils as green biopesticides: Recent global scenario. In: Essentials Oils. II. Recent Progress in Medicinal Plants. Vol. 37. USA: Studium Press LLC; 2013. pp. 151-218

[8] Khater HF. Prospects of botanical biopesticides in insect pest management. Pharmacologia. 2012; **3**(12):641-656

[9] Benelli G, Mehlhorn H. Declining malaria, rising of dengue and Zika virus: Insights for mosquito vector control. Parasitology Research. 2016;**115**(5): 1747-1754

[10] Benelli G. Research in mosquito control: Current challenges for a brighter future. Parasitology Research. 2015;**114**(8):2801-2805

[11] Khater H. Spice up your Life and Garden: Precious Treasures in your Kitchen. Washington: Kindle Direct Publisher; 2017. p. 135

[12] Moore SJ, Debboun M. History of insect repellents. In: Insect Repellents: Principles, Methods and Uses. Boca Raton, FL: CRC Press, Taylor & Francis group; 2007. pp. 3-29. Available from: https://books.google.com.eg/books?hl=ar&lr=&id=l2DLBQAAQBAJ&oi=fnd&pg=PA3&dq=Moore+SJ,+Debboun+M.+History+of+58+insect+repellents.+In:+Insect+Repellents:+59+Principles,+Methods+and+Uses.+2007.+60+pp.+3-29&ots=FCV6oMhPld&sig=qm12c7HUgu2uDMNS6ygQ6SXnHfY&redir_esc=y#v=onepage&q&f=false

[13] Islam J et al. Mosquito repellents: An insight into the chronological perspectives and novel discoveries. Acta Tropica. 2017;**167**(Suppl. C):216-230

[14] Lupi E, Hatz C, Schlagenhauf P. The efficacy of repellents against *Aedes*, *Anopheles*, *Culex* and *Ixodes* spp.—A literature review. Travel Medicine and Infectious Disease. 2013;**11**(6):374-411

[15] Yadav NP et al. A novel approach for development and characterization of effective mosquito repellent cream formulation containing citronella oil. BioMed Research International. 2014; **2014**:1-11. Available from: http://dx.doi.org/10.1155/2016/6475624

[16] Reiter P. Global warming and malaria: Knowing the horse before

hitching the cart. Malaria Journal. 2008; 7(1):S3

[17] Khater HF. Ecosmart biorational insecticides: Alternative insect control strategies. In: Insecticides—Advances in Integrated Pest Management. Rijeka, Croatia: InTech; 2012

[18] Pavela R, Benelli G. Ethnobotanical knowledge on botanical repellents employed in the African region against mosquito vectors—A review. Experimental Parasitology. 2016;**167** (Suppl. C):103-108

[19] Weldon PJ et al. Benzoquinones from millipedes deter mosquitoes and elicit self-anointing in capuchin monkeys (*Cebus* spp.). Naturwissenschaften. 2003;**90**(7): 301-304

[20] Pavela R, Benelli G. Essential oils as ecofriendly biopesticides? Challenges and constraints. Trends in Plant Science. 2016;**21**(12):1000-1007

[21] Norris EJ, Coats JR. Current and future repellent technologies: The potential of spatial repellents and their place in mosquito-borne disease control. International Journal of Environmental Research and Public Health. 2017;**14**(2): 124

[22] Leal WS. The enigmatic reception of DEET—The gold standard of insect repellents. Current Opinion in Insect Science. 2014;**6**:93-98

[23] Deletre E et al. Prospects for repellent in pest control: Current developments and future challenges. Chemoecology. 2016;**26**(4):127-142

[24] Boeckh J et al. Acylated 1,3-aminopropanols as repellents against bloodsucking arthropods. Pest Management Science. 1996;**48**(4): 359-373

[25] Pages F et al. Tick repellents for human use: Prevention of tick bites and tick-borne diseases. Vector Borne and Zoonotic Diseases. 2014;**14**(2):85-93

[26] Frances S et al. Field evaluation of repellent formulations containing deet and picaridin against mosquitoes in Northern Territory, Australia. Journal of Medical Entomology. 2004;**41**(3): 414-417

[27] Costantini C, Badolo A, Ilboudo-Sanogo E. Field evaluation of the efficacy and persistence of insect repellents DEET, IR3535, and KBR 3023 against *Anopheles gambiae* complex and other Afrotropical vector mosquitoes. Transactions of the Royal Society of Tropical Medicine and Hygiene. 2004; **98**(11):644-652

[28] Frances S et al. Field evaluation of commercial repellent formulations against mosquitoes (*Diptera*: *Culicidae*) in Northern Territory, Australia. Journal of the American Mosquito Control Association. 2005;**21**(4):480-482

[29] Goodyer L, Schofield S. Mosquito repellents for the traveller: Does picaridin provide longer protection than DEET?. Journal of Travel Medicine. 2018;**25**(Suppl_1):S10-S15

[30] Bissinger BW, Roe RM. Tick repellents: Past, present, and future. Pesticide Biochemistry and Physiology. 2010;**96**(2):63-79

[31] Nasci RS, Wirtz RA, Brogdon WG. Protection against mosquitoes, ticks, and other arthropods. In: CDC Health Information for International Travel. New York: Oxford University Press; 2016. pp. 94-99. Available from: https://books.google.com.eg/books?hl=ar&lr=&id=HshsCAAAQBAJ&oi=fnd&pg=PA94&dq=NASCI,+Roger+S.%3B+WIRTZ,+Robert+A.%3B+BROGDON,+William+G.+Protection+against+mosquitoes,+ticks,+and+other+arthropods.+CDC+health+information+for+international+travel,+2016,+94-9.%E2%80%8F&ots=rH6BQaUTl-&sig=

v5Ybtw5KXSO_D90cAxtN0hO23PI&redir_esc=y#v=onepage&q&f=false

[32] Carroll SP. Prolonged efficacy of IR3535 repellents against mosquitoes and blacklegged ticks in North America. Journal of Medical Entomology. 2008; **45**(4):706-714

[33] Kain P et al. Odour receptors and neurons for DEET and new insect repellents. Nature. 2013;**502**(7472):507

[34] Islam J et al. Protection against mosquito vectors *Aedes aegypti*, *Anopheles stephensi* and *Culex quinquefasciatus* using a novel insect repellent, ethyl anthranilate. Acta Tropica. 2017;**174**:56-63

[35] Isman MB et al. Essential Oil-Based Pesticides: New Insights from Old Chemistry. Weinheim, Germany: Wiley-VCH; 2007

[36] Vaz NP, De Oliveira DR, Abouelella GA, Khater H. In: Govil J, editor. The Black Seed, *Nigella sativa* (Ranunculaceae), For Prevention and Treatment of Hypertension. USA: Studium Press LLC.; 2018

[37] Seddiek SA et al. Anthelmintic activity of the white wormwood, *Artemisia herba-alba* against *Heterakis gallinarum* infecting Turkey poults. Journal of Medicinal Plant Research. 2011;**5**(16):3946-3957

[38] Nerio LS, Olivero-Verbel J, Stashenko E. Repellent activity of essential oils: A review. Bioresource Technology. 2010;**101**(1):372-378

[39] Maia MF, Moore SJ. Plant-based insect repellents: A review of their efficacy, development and testing. Malaria Journal. 2011;**10**(1):S11

[40] Batish DR et al. Eucalyptus essential oil as a natural pesticide. Forest Ecology and Management. 2008;**256**(12): 2166-2174

[41] Al-Quraishy S et al. Observations on effects of a neem seed extract (MiteStop®) on biting lice (mallophages) and bloodsucking insects parasitizing horses. Parasitology Research. 2012;**110**(1):335-339

[42] Khater HF, El-Shorbagy MM, Seddiek SA. Lousicidal efficacy of camphor oil, d-phenothrin, and deltamethrin against the slender pigeon louse, *Columbicola columbae*. International Journal of Veterinary Science and Medicine. 2014;**2**(1):7-13

[43] Khater HF. Bioactivities of some essential oils against the camel nasal botfly, *Cephalopina titillator*. Parasitology Research. 2014;**113**(2): 593-605

[44] Shalaby A, Khater H. Toxicity of certain solvent extracts of *Rosmarinus officinalis* against *Culex pipiens* larvae. Journal of Egyptian-German Society of Zoology E. 2005;**48**:69-80

[45] Khater HF, Shalaby AA-S. Potential of biologically active plant oils to control mosquito larvae (Culex pipiens, *Diptera: Culicidae*) from an Egyptian locality. Revista do Instituto de Medicina Tropical de São Paulo. 2008;**50**(2): 107-112

[46] Khater HF, Ramadan MY, Mageid ADA. In vitro control of the camel nasal botfly, *Cephalopina titillator*, with doramectin, lavender, camphor, and onion oils. Parasitology Research. 2013; **112**(7):2503-2510

[47] Khater HF, Ramadan MY, El-Madawy RS. Lousicidal, ovicidal and repellent efficacy of some essential oils against lice and flies infesting water buffaloes in Egypt. Veterinary Parasitology. 2009;**164**(2-4): 257-266

[48] Khater HF, Khater D. The insecticidal activity of four medicinal plants against the blowfly *Lucilia*

sericata (*Diptera*: *Calliphoridae*). International Journal of Dermatology. 2009;**48**(5):492-497

[49] Khater HF et al. Control of the myiasis-producing fly, *Lucilia sericata*, with Egyptian essential oils. International Journal of Dermatology. 2011;**50**(2):187-194

[50] Khater HF et al. Toxicity and growth inhibition potential of vetiver, cinnamon, and lavender essential oils and their blends against larvae of the sheep blowfly, *Lucilia sericata*. International Journal of Dermatology. 2018;**57**(4):449-457

[51] Krajick K. Keeping the bugs at bay. Science. 2006;**313**(5783):36-38. DOI: 10.1126/science.313.5783.36. Available from: https://science.sciencemag.org/content/313/5783/36?ijkey=2e16a3949e13d8253c2419859114f8dc92c569c2&keytype2=tf_ipsecsha

[52] Moore SJ, Mordue AJ, Logan JG. Insect bite prevention. Infectious Disease Clinics. 2012;**26**(3):655-673

[53] Vesin A et al. Transfluthrin indoor air concentration and inhalation exposure during application of electric vaporizers. Environment International. 2013;**60**:1-6

[54] Li H, Lydy MJ, You J. Pyrethroids in indoor air during application of various mosquito repellents: Occurrence, dissipation and potential exposure risk. Chemosphere. 2016;**144**:2427-2435

[55] Sengupta P, Banerjee R. Environmental toxins: Alarming impacts of pesticides on male fertility. Human & Experimental Toxicology. 2014;**33**(10):1017-1039

[56] Sinha C et al. Mosquito repellent (pyrethroid-based) induced dysfunction of blood-brain barrier permeability in developing brain. International Journal of Developmental Neuroscience. 2004; **22**(1):31-37

[57] Sinha C et al. Behavioral and neurochemical effects induced by pyrethroid-based mosquito repellent exposure in rat offsprings during prenatal and early postnatal period. Neurotoxicology and Teratology. 2006; **28**(4):472-481

[58] Bohlmann AM, Broschard T, Heider L. In: International Conference on Biopesticides VI; Chiang Mai, Thailand; 2011

[59] Meshram G, Rao K. N,N-diethylphenylacetamide, an insect repellent: Absence of mutagenic response in the in vitro Ames test and in vivo mouse micronucleus test. Food and Chemical Toxicology: An International Journal Published for the British Industrial Biological Research Association. 1988;**26**(9):791-796

[60] Rao S, Kaveeshwar U, Purkayastha S. Acute oral toxicity of insect repellent *N,N*-diethylphenylacetamide in mice, rats and rabbits and protective effect of sodium pentobarbital. Indian Journal of Experimental Biology. 1993;**31**(9): 755-760

[61] Rao S et al. Gas chromatographic identification of urinary metabolites of insect repellent *N,N*-diethylphenylacetamide on inhalation exposure in rats. Journal of Chromatography B: Biomedical Sciences and Applications. 1989;**493**:210-216

[62] Kline DL et al. Olfactometric evaluation of spatial repellents for *Aedes aegypti*. Journal of Medical Entomology. 2003;**40**(4):463-467

[63] Api A et al. RIFM fragrance ingredient safety assessment, ethyl anthranilate, CAS registry number 87-25-2. Food and Chemical Toxicology. 2015;**82**:S97-S104

[64] Manigrasso M et al. Temporal evolution of ultrafine particles and of alveolar deposited surface area from main indoor combustion and non-combustion sources in a model room. Science of the Total Environment. 2017; **598**:1015-1026

[65] Opdyke DLJ. Monographs on Fragrance Raw Materials. New York: First Pregamon Press; 1979

[66] Islam J et al. Exploration of ethyl anthranilate-loaded monolithic matrix-type prophylactic polymeric patch. Journal of Food and Drug Analysis. 2017;**25**(4):968-975

[67] Alpern JD et al. Personal protection measures against mosquitoes, ticks, and other arthropods. Medical Clinics. 2016; **100**(2):303-316

[68] Belščak-Cvitanović A, Durgo K, Huđek A, Bačun-Družina V, Komes D. Overview of polyphenols and their properties. In: Polyphenols: Properties, Recovery, and Applications. Woodhead Publishing; 2018. pp. 3-44. Available from: https://www.sciencedirect.com/science/article/pii/B9780128135723000014

[69] Mileo AM, Miccadei S. Polyphenols as modulator of oxidative stress in cancer disease: New therapeutic strategies. Oxidative Medicine and Cellular Longevity. 2016;**2016**:1-17. Article ID: 6475624. Available from: http://dx.doi.org/10.1155/2016/6475624

[70] Stanczyk NM et al. Behavioral insensitivity to DEET in *Aedes aegypti* is a genetically determined trait residing in changes in sensillum function. Proceedings of the National Academy of Sciences. 2010;**107**(19):8575-8580

[71] Klun JA et al. Comparative resistance of *Anopheles albimanus* and *Aedes aegypti* to N,N-diethyl-3-methylbenzamide (Deet) and 2-methylpiperidinyl-3-cyclohexen-1-carboxamide (AI3-37220) in laboratory human-volunteer repellent assays. Journal of Medical Entomology. 2004; **41**(3):418-422

[72] Murugan K et al. Predation by Asian bullfrog tadpoles, *Hoplobatrachus tigerinus*, against the dengue vector, *Aedes aegypti*, in an aquatic environment treated with mosquitocidal nanoparticles. Parasitology Research. 2015;**114**(10):3601-3610

[73] Roni M et al. Characterization and biotoxicity of *Hypnea* musciformis-synthesized silver nanoparticles as potential eco-friendly control tool against *Aedes aegypti* and *Plutella xylostella*. Ecotoxicology and Environmental Safety. 2015;**121**:31-38

[74] Govindarajan M et al. One-pot fabrication of silver nanocrystals using *Nicandra* physalodes: A novel route for mosquito vector control with moderate toxicity on non-target water bugs. Research in Veterinary Science. 2016; **107**:95-101

[75] Govindarajan M et al. Single-step biosynthesis and characterization of silver nanoparticles using *Zornia diphylla* leaves: A potent eco-friendly tool against malaria and arbovirus vectors. Journal of Photochemistry and Photobiology B: Biology. 2016;**161**: 482-489

[76] Benelli G et al. Mosquito control with green nanopesticides: Towards the one health approach? A review of non-target effects. Environmental Science and Pollution Research. 2018;**25**(11): 10184-10206

[77] Balaji APB et al. Polymeric nanoencapsulation of insect repellent: Evaluation of its bioefficacy on *Culex quinquefasciatus* mosquito population and effective impregnation onto cotton fabrics for insect repellent clothing.

Journal of King Saud University—Science. 2017;**29**(4):517-527

[78] Karr JI, Speaker TJ, Kasting GB. A novel encapsulation of *N,N*-diethyl-3-methylbenzamide (DEET) favorably modifies skin absorption while maintaining effective evaporation rates. Journal of Controlled Release. 2012; **160**(3):502-508

[79] Nogueira Barradas T et al. Polymer-based drug delivery systems applied to insects repellents devices: A review. Current Drug Delivery. 2016;**13**(2): 221-235

[80] Misni N, Nor ZM, Ahmad R. Repellent effect of microencapsulated essential oil in lotion formulation against mosquito bites. Journal of Vector Borne Diseases. 2017;**54**(1):44

[81] Solomon B et al. Microencapsulation of citronella oil for mosquito-repellent application: Formulation and in vitro permeation studies. European Journal of Pharmaceutics and Biopharmaceutics. 2012;**80**(1):61-66

[82] Ribeiro AD et al. Microencapsulation of citronella oil for solar-activated controlled release as an insect repellent. Applied Materials Today. 2016;**5**:90-97

[83] Leal WS. Molecular-based chemical prospecting of mosquito attractants and repellents. In: Insect Repellents: Principles, Methods, and Uses. Boca Raton: CRC Press; 2007. pp. 229-242

[84] Tauxe GM et al. Targeting a dual detector of skin and CO_2 to modify mosquito host seeking. Cell. 2013; **155**(6):1365-1379

[85] Govere J et al. Efficacy of three insect repellents against the malaria vector *Anopheles arabiensis*. Medical and Veterinary Entomology. 2000;**14**(4): 441-444

[86] Witting-Bissinger B et al. Novel arthropod repellent, BioUD, is an efficacious alternative to deet. Journal of Medical Entomology. 2008;**45**(5): 891-898

[87] Barnard DR, Xue R-D. Laboratory evaluation of mosquito repellents against *Aedes albopictus*, *Culex nigripalpus*, and *Ochlerotatus triseriatus* (*Diptera*: *Culicidae*). Journal of Medical Entomology. 2004;**41**(4):726-730

[88] Webb CE, Russell RC. Is the extract from the plant catmint (*Nepeta cataria*) repellent to mosquitoes in Australia? Journal of the American Mosquito Control Association. 2007;**23**(3):351-354

[89] Lindsay LR et al. Evaluation of the efficacy of 3Vo citronella candles and 5Vo citronella incense for protection against field populations of *Aedes* mosquitoes. Journal of the American Mosquito Control Association. 1996;**12**: 293-294

[90] Fradin MS, Day JF. Comparative efficacy of insect repellents against mosquito bites. New England Journal of Medicine. 2002;**347**(1):13-18

[91] Tuetun B et al. Repellent properties of celery, *Apium graveolens* L., compared with commercial repellents, against mosquitoes under laboratory and field conditions. Tropical Medicine & International Health. 2005;**10**(11): 1190-1198

[92] Tuetun B et al. Celery-based topical repellents as a potential natural alternative for personal protection against mosquitoes. Parasitology Research. 2008;**104**(1):107-115

[93] Chang KS et al. Repellency of cinnamomum cassia bark compounds and cream containing cassia oil to *Aedes aegypti* (*Diptera*: *Culicidae*) under laboratory and indoor conditions. Pest Management Science. 2006;**62**(11): 1032-1038

[94] Kim SI et al. Repellency of aerosol and cream products containing fennel oil to mosquitoes under laboratory and field conditions. Pest Management Science. 2004;**60**(11):1125-1130

[95] Trongtokit Y, Curtis CF, Rongsriyam Y. Efficacy of repellent products against caged and free flying *Anopheles stephensi* mosquitoes. Southeast Asian Journal of Tropical Medicine and Public Health. 2005;**36**(6):1423

[96] Mittal P et al. Efficacy of advanced odomos repellent cream (*N*,*N*-diethyl-benzamide) against mosquito vectors. The Indian Journal of Medical Research. 2011;**133**(4):426

[97] McPhatter LP, Mischler PD, Webb MZ, Chauhan K, Lindroth EJ, Richardson AG, et al. Laboratory and semi-field evaluations of two (Transfluthrin) spatial repellent devices against *Aedes aeǵypti* (L.) (*Diptera*: *Culicidae*). US Army Medical Department Journal. January-June 2017, pp.13-22. Available from: https://www.researchgate.net/profile/Lee_Mcphatter/publication/323016579_Laboratory_and_semi-field_evaluations_of_two_transfluthrin_spatial_repellent_devices_against_Aedes_aegypti_L_Diptera_Culicidae/links/5b7ef0f74585151fd12e6481/Laboratory-and-semi-field-evaluations-of-two-transfluthrin-spatial-repellent-devices-against-Aedes-aegypti-L-Diptera-Culicidae.pdf#page=15

[98] Lucas J et al. US Laboratory and field trials of metofluthrin (SumiOne®) emanators for reducing mosquito biting outdoors. Journal of the American Mosquito Control Association. 2007;**23**(1):47-54

[99] Xue R-D et al. Field evaluation of the off! Clip-on mosquito repellent (metofluthrin) against *Aedes albopictus* and *Aedes taeniorhynchus* (Diptera: Culicidae) in northeastern Florida. Journal of Medical Entomology. 2012;**49**(3):652-655

[100] Dame DA et al. Field evaluation of four spatial repellent devices against Arkansas rice-land mosquitoes. Journal of the American Mosquito Control Association. 2014;**30**(1):31-36